1991-1992

Pocketbook of Pediatric Antimicrobial Therapy

NINTH EDITION

John D. Nelson, M.D.

Professor of Pediatrics
The University of Texas
Southwestern Medical Center at Dallas
Southwestern Medical School
Dallas, Texas

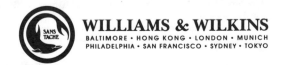

WILLIAMS & WILKINS
BALTIMORE · HONG KONG · LONDON · MUNICH
PHILADELPHIA · SAN FRANCISCO · SYDNEY · TOKYO

*The mention of a product name does
not imply endorsement by the author.*

Editor: Laurel Craven
Associate Editor: Victoria M. Vaughn
Copy Editor: Clifford L. Malanowski, Jr.
Designer: Dan Pfisterer
Production Coordinator: Barbara J. Felton

Copyright © 1991
Williams & Wilkins
428 East Preston Street
Baltimore, Maryland 21202, USA

Accurate indications, adverse reactions, and dosage schedules for drugs are provided in this book, but it is possible that they may change. The reader is urged to review the package information data of the manufacturers of the medications mentioned.

Printed in the United States of America

Library of Congress Cataloging in Publication Data

Nelson, John D., 1930-
    1991-1992 Pocketbook of pediatric antimicrobial therapy/John D. Nelson. — 9th ed.
       p. cm.
    Rev. ed. of: Pocketbook of pediatric antimicrobial therapy. [1975]
    Includes index.
      1. Communicable diseases in children — Chemotherapy — Handbooks, manuals, etc. 2. Antibiotics — Handbooks, manuals, etc. I. Nelson, John D., 1930- . Pocketbook of pediatric antimicrobial therapy. II. Title.
     [DNLM: 1. Antibiotics — therapeutic use — handbooks. 2. Drug Therapy — in infancy & childhood — handbooks. QV 39 N427p]
RJ53.A5N44 1989   615.5′8 — dc19   88-26186
    ISBN 0-683-06404-5

                        90 91 92 93 94
             1 2 3 4 5 6 7 8 9 10

CONTENTS

I. INTRODUCTION TO THE NINTH EDITION

This book is revised every 2 years and generally I am astonished at the number of new antimicrobials marketed. For the previous edition there had been 11 new agents during the preceding 2 years. Not so this time. The flood of new cephalosporins appears to have abated--at least temporarily. Only one new cephalosporin was marketed during the past 2 years. That was cefixime (Suprax®) which was actually included in the previous edition because I knew its release was imminent at that time.

There have been four new antimicrobials. One is mefloquine (Lariam®), an anti-malarial drug used in adults for prophylaxis or treatment, including chloroquine resistant *Plasmodium falciparum*. It is not presently approved for use in children because of unacceptably high rates of gastrointestinal side effects.

The other three drugs reflect the changing world of modern medicine: human immunodeficiency virus infected patients, organ transplant patients and other immunosuppressed children who fill the beds of tertiary care hospitals. Dideoxyinosine (Videx®) is used exclusively for suppression of HIV infection. It is still being evaluated in clinical protocols but it is available for patients who cannot take zidovudine (AZT, Retrovir®).

Ganciclovir (Cytovene®), an analogue of acyclovir, has greater activity against cytomegalovirus than acyclovir. It is approved for treatment of CMV retinitis in immunocompromised patients but it is being used for treatment of CMV infections in other organs as well.

Fluconazole (Diflucan®) is an antifungal agent available for intravenous or oral use. It is approved for treatment of cryptococcal meningitis and systemic *Candida* infections. It has excellent penetration into cerebrospinal fluid and it is well tolerated with few side effects. It is possible that it will be used in other types of fungal infection since it has good activity against several other fungi.

The experience with the many new antimicrobials of recent vintage has necessitated extensive revision of the **Pocketbook**. The large numbers of related drugs mean that multiple options are available for a great many diseases. To avoid cluttering up and expanding the **Pocketbook** I have indicated only one or two options for treating most infections. Clearly, other regimens might be suitable.

Some dosages and indications differ from those in the manufacturers' package inserts. In such situations the dosages recommended in this book have been found by controlled studies or by clinical experience to be efficacious and safe.

The continued popularity and apparent utility of this little book is gratifying. As in the past, I encourage you to send suggestions for its improvement to me.

John D. Nelson, M.D.

Department of Pediatrics
The University of Texas
Southwestern Medical Center at Dallas
5323 Harry Hines Blvd.
Dallas, Texas 75235

II. CHOOSING AMONG AMINOGLYCOSIDES, CEPHALOSPORINS AND PENICILLINS

New drugs should be compared with others in the same class regarding (1) antimicrobial spectrum, (2) degree of potency within the spectrum, (3) pharmacokinetic properties, (4) demonstrated efficacy in clinical trials, (5) tolerance, toxicity and side effects, and (6) cost. If there is no substantial benefit in any of those areas, one should opt for staying with the older, familiar drug because of the risk of unexpected adverse effects inherent in any new product.

Aminoglycosides. Five aminoglycosidic antibiotics are available in the U.S. as major drugs for coliform bacillary infections: amikacin, gentamicin, kanamycin, netilmicin and tobramycin. (Streptomycin and spectinomycin are seldom used.) Amikacin is likely to be effective against coliform bacilli resistant to the other four agents. For this reason, when it was first released it was reserved for treatment of infections caused by multiply-resistant organisms; however, emergence of resistance has not been a problem in several hospitals in which it has been used almost exclusively for several years. Kanamycin is not effective against *Pseudomonas aeruginosa* so the others are preferred whenever that infection is present or suspected. There are small differences in comparative toxicities of these aminoglycosides to the kidneys and eighth cranial nerve. In animal models netilmicin is the least toxic. It is possible that netilmicin and tobramycin are the safest, but there are conflicting reports in studies focusing on small changes in renal function rather than frank renal failure. It is uncertain whether or not these small differences are clinically significant. In any case, it is advisable to monitor peak and trough serum concentrations in all patients; elevated peak and trough concentrations correlate with toxicity. Desired peak concentrations with amikacin and kanamycin are 20-35 μg/ml and trough concentrations less than 10 μg/ml; for the others they are 5-10 μg/ml and less than 2 μg/ml, respectively. Patients with cystic fibrosis require larger than normal dosage to achieve therapeutic serum concentrations and they excrete aminoglycosides more rapidly. In the case of nosocomial infection, the choice among aminoglycosides should be based on knowledge of local susceptibility patterns. In addition to routine monitoring of *in vitro* susceptibility testing results to detect emergence of resistant strains, the policy of switching among the drugs for routine hospital use every one to two years might minimize the likelihood of resistance due to selective drug pressure.

Oral Cephalosporins (Cefaclor, cefadroxil, cefixime, cefuroxime axetil, cephalexin and cephradine). As a class, the oral cephalosporins have the advantages over oral penicillins of somewhat greater safety and greater palatability of the suspension formulations. (Penicillins have a bitter taste.) Cefuroxime is the least palatable. They have the disadvantage of being more expensive than penicillin derivatives. Cephalexin and cephradine have virtually identical properties and effectiveness and can be used interchangeably. The half-life of cefadroxil in serum is about twice as long as that of the other drugs. This pharmacokinetic feature accounts for the fact that cefadroxil can be given in only one or two daily doses. Cefaclor, cefixime and cefuroxime have the advantage of adding *Haemophilus influenzae* (including beta-lactamase producing strains) to the spectrum. Cefixime is unique in this group in having no useful activity against staphylococci.

Parenteral Cephalosporins. First generation cephalosporins (cefazolin, cephalothin, cephapirin, cephradine) have limited application in pediatrics. They have been used mainly as back-up drugs for treatment of Gram-positive infections because their Gram-negative spectrum is limited. Cefazolin is tolerated best on intramuscular injection; furthermore, it is given q8h because of its longer half-life in serum rather than the q4-6h schedules used for the others. Differences in the frequencies of vein irritation among the group are minor.

The second generation cephalosporins (cefamandole and cefuroxime) and the cephamycin (cefoxitin) added to the antibacterial spectrum. Cefoxitin has good activity against *B. fragilis* and can be used in place of chloramphenicol or clindamycin when that organism is implicated in disease. Cefotetan has a spectrum similar to that of cefoxitin but a longer serum half-life, so it can be given q12h. Cefamandole and cefuroxime added *Haemophilus influenzae* to the spectrum of cephalosporins. However, cefamandole is somewhat unstable to the TEM1 beta-lactamase elaborated by *H. influenzae*. This combined with its rather poor penetration into cerebrospinal fluid has resulted in cases of *Haemophilus* meningitis developing in infants being treated with cefamandole. Cefuroxime is more stable to the enzyme and has better penetration into CSF (comparable to that of ampicillin). It has been used to treat meningitis due to the usual pathogens. Cefuroxime has utility as single drug therapy (in place of combinations such as nafcillin and chloramphenicol) for infants and young children with pneumonia, bone and joint infections or other conditions in which Gram-positive cocci and *Haemophilus* are the usual pathogens. Two related drugs, ceforanide and cefonicid, were released for use in 1984. They differ in having prolonged serum half-lives so that doses can be given every 12 to 24 hours. Cefonicid is not yet approved for use in children. Ceforanide has limited activity against some strains of *Haemophilus*; I believe that it has no role in Pediatrics.

Among the many so-called third generation cephalosporins, cefoperazone is not yet approved for use in children. (Moxalactam is technically an oxacephem rather than a cephalosporin.) All have enhanced potency against many Gram-negative bacilli, usually including aminoglycoside resistant organisms. They are inactive against enterococci and *Listeria* and have variable activity against *Pseudomonas* and *Bacteroides*. Moxalactam has poorer activity than the others against Gram-positive cocci. Cefotaxime and ceftriaxone have been used successfully to treat meningitis due to the usual pathogens, and moxalactam is effective for coliform and *Haemophilus* (but not pneumococcal) meningitis. Limited experience with ceftazidime and ceftizoxime suggests they too are effective for meningitis. These drugs have greatest utility for treating Gram-negative bacillary infections when aminoglycosides are contraindicated or when the organisms are resistant to customarily used drugs. Because cefoperazone and ceftriaxone are excreted to a large extent via the liver, they can be used with little dosage adjustment in patients with renal failure. Ceftazidime has the unique property of activity against *Pseudomonas aeruginosa* that is comparable to that of the

3

aminoglycosides. Ceftriaxone has a serum half-life of 4 to 7 hours and can be given once or twice a day.

Penicillinase-resistant Penicillins (Cloxacillin, dicloxacillin, methicillin, nafcillin, oxacillin). Nafcillin differs pharmacologically from the others in being excreted primarily by the liver rather than by the kidneys. This may be the reason for its lack of nephrotoxicity. Nephrotoxicity or hemorrhagic cystitis occurs in 5% of children treated with methicillin. For this reason nafcillin is preferred over methicillin or oxacillin for parenteral use with two exceptions: the neonate and patients with hepatic disease. Nafcillin pharmacokinetics in the newborn are erratic, especially in jaundiced babies; furthermore, methicillin nephrotoxicity is rare in the neonate. Although nafcillin is not known to aggravate pre-existing hepatic disease, it seems prudent to avoid a drug that is highly concentrated in the liver in those circumstances. For oral use, cloxacillin, oxacillin and dicloxacillin are essentially equivalent but the latter has greater anti-staphylococcal activity *in vitro*.

Anti-pseudomonas Penicillins (Azlocillin, carbenicillin, imipenem, mezlocillin, piperacillin, ticarcillin, ticarcillin-clavulanate). Ticarcillin and mezlocillin are quantitatively more effective against *Pseudomonas aeruginosa* than is carbenicillin. Azlocillin and piperacillin are the most active *in vitro* against *Pseudomonas*. Carbenicillin has a much greater sodium content than the other drugs. Mezlocillin does not affect platelet adhesiveness significantly but the others do; this could be an advantage in patients who have another risk factor for bleeding. In general, *Pseudomonas* strains resistant to ticarcillin are resistant to the newer drugs. These drugs should be used along with an aminoglycoside or cephalosporin for treating *Pseudomonas* infections in compromised hosts for synergistic effect. Timentin® is the combination of ticarcillin and the beta-lactamase inhibitor, clavulanate. The combination has little effect on activity against *Pseudomonas* but does extend the spectrum to many beta-lactamase-positive bacteria. Imipenem is a carbapenem with a broader spectrum of activity than any other beta-lactam currently available. It is not approved by the FDA for use in children and experience is limited. At present it is recommended for treatment of infections caused by *Pseudomonas* and other bacteria resistant to all other drugs.

Aminopenicillins (Amoxicillin, amoxicillin-clavulanate, ampicillin, ampicillin-sulbactam, bacampicillin, cyclacillin). Bacampicillin is rapidly and completely converted in the body to ampicillin so it is an indirect means of administering ampicillin. Bacampicillin and cyclacillin are the most efficiently absorbed so peak blood levels are greater than after the same dosage of amoxicillin or ampicillin. Ampicillin is more likely than the others to cause diarrhea and to disturb colonic coliform flora and cause overgrowth of Candida. Augmentin® is a combination of amoxicillin and clavulanate for oral use that permits amoxicillin to be active against beta-lactamase-producing bacteria (but not *Pseudomonas*). Sulbactam, another beta-lactamase inhibitor, is combined with ampicillin in the parenteral formulation, Unasyn®. Clinical experience is too limited to date to assess its role in pediatric patients.

4

Monobactams. The only monobactam licensed for use in the U.S. is aztreonam. Its spectrum is similar to that of the anti-*Pseudomonas* aminoglycosides so the clinical indications are similar. Experience with the drug to date is insufficient to know for which clinical situations, if any, that it might replace the aminoglycosides.

III. PENICILLIN DESENSITIZATION

Studies have shown that an oral regimen is safer and more effective than graduated injections for desensitization to penicillins. (**Pediatr Infect Dis** 1:344, 1982)

Penicillin V suspension is used. Signed, informed consent is recommended. An intravenous line is in place and emergency resuscitation materials at hand for the unlikely event of anaphylaxis. A physician should be in attendance. Doses are given at 15 minute intervals; the total regimen requires 4 hours.

Doses	Penicillin V units/ml	Amount q15 min
#1-#7	1,000	Doubling doses from 0.1 ml (100 units) to 6.4 ml (6,400 units)
#8-#10	10,000	Doubling doses from 1.2 ml (12,000 units) to 4.8 ml (48,000 units)
#11-#14	80,000	Doubling doses from 1.0 ml (80,000 units) to 8.0 ml (640,000 units)

(Reference: **New Engl J Med** 1985;312:1229)

Minor allergic reactions are suppressed with epinephrine or antihistamines. Therapy is not interrupted unless there is a severe or unsuppressible reaction. If there are interruptions in therapy of more than 8 hours, it is advisable to repeat the desensitization regimen.

If the patient cannot tolerate oral medication, parenteral desensitization can be used. The method is reviewed in **J Allergy Clin Immunol** 69:275, 1982.

IV. SEQUENTIAL PARENTERAL-ORAL ANTIBIOTIC THERAPY FOR SERIOUS INFECTIONS

Bacterial pneumonias, endocarditis and bone and joint infections often require prolonged antibiotic therapy. Intravenous therapy not only is unpleasant for the child but carries a hazard of serious nosocomial disease.

Rationale:
1. Comparable dosages of analogous parenteral and oral medications result in comparable serum concentrations from 1-6 hours after a dose and comparable bioavailability ("area-under-the-curve") in most patients.
2. There is no known therapeutic advantage to the momentary high serum concentrations during IV administration.
3. Although the protein binding of many oral formulations is greater than that of parenteral formulations, this does not prevent good penetration into body fluid compartments.

Method:
1. Initial parenteral therapy
   a. Alert laboratory to save pathogen for serum bactericidal tests. (Serum bactericidal titer 1-2 hours after an IV dose for baseline value is optional.
   b. Perform any necessary surgical procedures.
2. Subsequent oral therapy when clinical condition is stable and patient is able to take and retain oral medication
   a. Select appropriate oral antibiotic based on *in vitro* susceptibilities and compliance factors (mainly palatability of suspension formulations).
   b. BEGIN WITH DOSAGE 2-3 TIMES "NORMAL" DOSAGE: e.g. 75-100 MG/KG/DAY OF DICLOXACILLIN AND 100-150 MG/KG/DAY OF OTHER BETA-LACTAMS.
   c. Serum bactericidal titer 1-2 hours after a dose.
   d. Adjust dosage if titer not at least 1:8.

NOTES:
1. The serum bactericidal titer is done quantitatively and is defined as ≥ 99.9% killing (100% killing is seldom achieved). For staphylococcal or *Haemophilus* infections the serum bactericidal titer should be at least 1:8. For highly susceptible bacteria such as pneumococci and Group A streptococci, titers are usually greater than 1:32.
2. Peak serum activity usually is found 45 to 60 minutes after a dose taken as suspension and 1-2 hours after a capsule or tablet.
3. These large dosages are surprisingly well-tolerated and gastrointestinal side effects are rare.
4. Approximately 5-10% of patients are unsuitable for this regimen because of poor GI absorption of antibiotics.

WARNING: ORAL THERAPY REGIMENS FOR SERIOUS INFECTIONS ARE POTENTIALLY HAZARDOUS UNLESS ADEQUACY OF SERUM BACTERICIDAL ACTIVITY IS MONITORED.

V. ANTIBIOTIC THERAPY FOR NEWBORNS

A. RECOMMENDED THERAPY FOR SELECTED CONDITIONS

NOTE: To avoid repetition, the recommended dosages and intervals of administration of antibiotics indicated with an asterisk in most of the following conditions are given in the Table on pages 16 and 17.

Condition	Therapy	Comment
Congenital syphilis	Penicillin G 100,000-150,000 u/kg day IV div q8-12h OR procaine penicillin G 50,000 u/kg/day IM div q24h x 10-14 days; (? 21 days for CNS disease)	Obtain follow-up serology at 3,6,12 mos
Congenital toxoplasmosis	Trisulfapyrimidines or sulfadiazine 85 mg/kg/day PO div q6h AND pyrimethamine 1 mg/kg PO once daily x 6 mos.; Steroids for chorioretinitis; FOLLOWED BY: spiramycin (available from CDC) 100 mg/kg/day PO div q12h given subsequently in alternating courses of 1 month each with pyrimethamine and sulfa x 6 mos.	Supplemental folinic acid 5 mg every 3 days; See Remington and Klein, **Infectious Diseases of the Fetus and Newborn Infant,** 3rd ed, for detailed recommendations
Herpes simplex infection	Acyclovir 30 mg/kg/day as 1-2 hr IV infusion div q8h OR vidarabine 15-30 mg/kg/day as 12 hour or longer IV infusion x 10 days; PLUS trifluoridine ophthalmic sol'n q2h for conjunctivitis	Larger dosage of vidarabine may prevent dissemination of skin disease
Tetanus neonatorum	Penicillin G* IV x 10 days	Antitoxin and sedation; Do not use IM injections
Parotitis, suppurative	Methicillin* IV AND aminoglycoside IV, IM x 10 days	Usually staphylococcal but occasionally coliform

8

Conjunctivitis
- Chlamydial

Erythromycin* estolate or ethylsuccinate PO x 10-14 days OR topical erythromycin, tetracycline or sulfacetamide ointment q.i.d.

Erythro PO preferable to topical therapy because NP carrier state eradicated; Treat mother and her sexual partner with tetracycline

- Gonococcal

Ceftriaxone 25-50 mg/kg/day (max. 125mg) IV, IM once daily OR cefotaxime 50 mg/kg/day IV, IM div q12h; x 7 days (A single dose of ceftriaxone may be effective in uncomplicated infection)

Chloramphenicol or tetra-cycline ophthalmic drops or ointment optional but not necessary; Treat mother and her sexual partner

- Staphylococcus aureus

Methicillin* IM, IV x 7-10 days

Additionally: Neomycin ophthalmic drops or ointment (systemic antibiotic not used for minor infection)

- Pseudomonas aeruginosa

Ticarcillin* or mezlocillin* IV, IM AND amino-glycoside* IM, IV x 7-10 days (Alternative: Ceftazidime*)

Polymyxin B ophthalmic drops or ointment; Subtenon or subconjunctival antibiotics in some cases

Gastrointestinal Infections
- Enteropathogenic E. coli

Neomycin 100 mg/kg/day PO div q8h x 5 days OR colistin 10-15 mg/kg/day PO div q8h x 5 days

Drugs effective in control-ling nosocomial spread; Most "enteropathogenic" strains neither toxigenic nor invasive

- Salmonella

Ampicillin* IM, IV x 7-10 days if suspected sepsis or focal infection; No antibiotic for uncomplicated gastroenteritis if self-limited

Observe for focal complications (meningitis, arthritis, etc.)

* See pages 16-17 for dosage

NEWBORN

9

NEWBORN

Condition	Therapy	Comment
- Necrotizing enterocolitis or peritonitis secondary to bowel rupture	Ticarcillin* IV, IM AND aminoglycoside* IM, IV x 10 days or longer; cefotaxime* suitable alternative to aminoglycoside; vancomycin* IV if S. epidermidis or methicillin-resistant staphylococcus cultured; common alternative: vancomycin* + clindamycin*	Bacteremia in 30-50% of cases; after 2-3 days of age Bacteroides common in gut; clindamycin* or metronidazole* for ticarcillin-resistant B. fragilis
Sepsis and Meningitis	NOTE: Dexamethasone adjunctive therapy for meningitis is currently being evaluated in neonates	
- Initial therapy	Ampicillin* or penicillin G* IV AND aminoglycoside* IV, IM	Duration of therapy: 7-10 days for sepsis without a focus; 21 days minimum for meningitis
		Ampicillin* AND cefotaxime* is a suitable alternative, especially if aminoglycoside-resistant nosocomial organism suspected
- Bacteroides fragilis ssp. fragilis	Metronidazole*, clindamycin*, mezlocillin* or ticarcillin* IV, IM	Metronidazole preferred for CNS infection
- Coliform bacteria	Cefotaxime* IV,IM; lumbar intrathecal or intraventricular injections of aminoglycoside are not beneficial in usual case	Aminoglycoside* is suitable alternative
- Group A or non-enterococcal Group D streptococci	Penicillin G* IV	
- Group B streptococcus	Ampicillin* or penicillin G* AND gentamicin IV, IM (Discontinue gentamicin when strain known to be fully susceptible to ampicillin)	Synergy may be advantage esp. against penicillin-tolerant strains
- Gonococcal	Ceftriaxone 25-50 mg/kg/day IV, IM once daily OR cefotaxime 50 mg/kg/day IV, IM div q12h	Penicillin G* for susceptible strains

10

- Listeria monocytogenes and enterococc.	Ampicillin* IV, IM AND aminoglycoside* IV, IM	Aminoglycosides synergistic in vitro with ampicillin
- Staphylococcus epidermidis	Vancomycin* IV, IM	Many methicillin-resistant
- Staphylococcus aureus	Methicillin* IV, IM; vancomycin* IV for methicillin-resistant Staphylococcus	Rarely causes meningitis in newborn; vancomycin preferred for meningitis
- Pseudomonas aeruginosa	Mezlocillin* or ticarcillin* IV, IM AND aminoglycoside* IV, IM	Ceftazidime* is a suitable alternative

Osteomyelitis, Suppurative Arthritis

Surgical drainage of pus; early institution of physical therapy

- Gonococcal arthritis and tenosynovitis	Ceftriaxone* IV, IM x 7-10 days (penicillin G* IV if organism susceptible)	
- Staphylococcus aureus	Methicillin* IV, IM x 21 days minimum; vancomycin* IV for methicillin-resistant Staphylococcus	Change to penicillin G if organism susceptible
- Coliform bacteria	Cefotaxime* OR aminoglycoside* IV, IM x 21 days minimum	Cephalosporins better than aminoglycosides for deep tissue infection
- Group B streptococcus	(See Group B streptococcal meningitis)	
- Unknown	Methicillin* IV, IM AND cefotaxime* IV, IM x 21 days minimum	

* See pages 16-17 for dosage

NEWBORN

Condition	Therapy	Comment
Otitis Media	Few controlled treatment trials in newborns; Suggest using initial therapy as for older infants (see page 24); If no response, obtain middle ear fluid for culture	Cefaclor or Augmentin may have advantage because of activity vs. coliforms and Staph. which cause disease in 10-20% of cases
- Coliform bacteria	Cefaclor 30-40 mg/kg/day PO div q8-12h x 10 days OR Augmentin (same dosage)	Aminoglycoside* or cefotaxime* if parenteral therapy needed
- *Staphylococcus aureus*	Cloxacillin 50 mg/kg/day PO div q6-8h x 10 days	Methicillin* if unable to treat PO
- Streptococcus (incl. pneumococcus)	Penicillin V 30 mg/kg/day PO div q8h x 10 days	Given IV, IM for complicated otitis
- *Haemophilus*	Cefaclor 30-40 mg/kg/day PO div q8-12h OR amoxicillin 30-40 mg/kg/day PO div q8-12h if susceptible	Other regimens not tested in neonates
Pulmonary Infections		
- *Staphylococcus aureus*	Methicillin* IV, IM x 21 days minimum; vancomycin* IV for methicillin-resistant Staph	Closed tube drainage of empyema
- *Pseudomonas aeruginosa*	Mezlocillin* or ticarcillin* IV, IM AND gentamicin* or amikacin* IV, IM x 14 days or longer	Ceftazidime* is a suitable alternative
- Group B streptococcus	Penicillin G* IV OR ampicillin* IV, IM x 10-14 days	Radiograph often mimics hyaline membrane disease
- *Chlamydia trachomatis*	Erythromycin* PO x 14-21 days	Ampicillin, amoxicillin or sulfa drugs may be effective
- *Pneumocystis carinii*	(See page 56)	

Condition	Treatment	Notes
- Aspiration pneumonia	Methicillin* IV, IM AND aminoglycoside* IV, IM x 7-10 days	Most aspiration episodes are not followed by pneumonia and do not require antibiotic therapy
- Pertussis	Erythromycin* x 5-10 days OR ampicillin* IV, IM if PO meds not retained	Usually acquired from parent or other adult in household
Skin and Soft Tissues - Impetigo neonatorum	Cleansing alone OR methicillin* IV, IM OR cephalexin 50 mg/kg/day PO div q6-8h x 5 days	No antibiotic for superficial impetigo; Hexachlorophene baths; Break lesions with alcohol swab
- Erysipelas (and other Group A streptococcal infections)	Penicillin G* IV x 5-7 days	Group B streptococcus may produce similar cellulitis or nodular lesions
- Breast abscess	Methicillin* IV, IM x 5-7 days; aminoglycoside* OR cefotaxime* if Gram-negative rods seen in pus	Gram stain of expressed pus/colostrum or I&D material necessary to select initial therapy; I&D of pus (Avoid damage to breast tissue)
- *Staphylococcus*	Methicillin* IV, IM x 5-7 days; vancomycin* for methicillin resistant *Staphylococcus*	Value of systemic antibiotics over surgical drainage alone not established
- Group B streptococcus	Penicillin G* IV OR ampicillin* IV, IM x 5-7 days	Usually no pus formed
- Coliform bacteria	Aminoglycoside* IM, IV x 5-7 days; Alternative: cefotaxime*	

* See pages 16-17 for dosage

13

NEWBORN

Condition	Therapy	Comment
Skin and Soft Tissues (cont.) - Omphalitis and Funisitis		
Group A or B streptococci	Penicillin G* IV x 5-7 days OR (for Group A strep) benzathine penicillin G 50,000 u/kg IM x 1 dose PLUS topical "triple dye" or bacitracin ointment	Group A strep usually causes "wet cord" without pus and with minimal erythema
Staphylococcus aureus	Methicillin* IV, IM x 5 days or longer	Observe for bacteremia and other focus of infection
Necrotizing funisitis	Methicillin* IV, IM AND aminoglycoside* IV, IM	Unknown etiology but coliform or staphylococcal secondary infection may occur
Clostridial	Penicillin G* IV x 10 days or longer	Crepitance and rapidly spreading cellulitis around umbilicus
Urinary Tract Infection		LARGER DOSAGES OF DRUGS REQUIRED IF ACCOMPANYING SEPSIS: Investigate for anomalies of urinary tract
- Coliform bacteria	Gentamicin 3 mg/kg/day IV, IM div q12h OR amikacin 10 mg/kg/day IV, IM div q12h x 10 days	Ampicillin used for *P. mirabilis* infection
- *Pseudomonas aeruginosa*	Mezlocillin or ticarcillin IV, IM 75-100 mg/kg/day IV, IM div q8-12h	Ceftazidime* is a suitable alternative
- Enterococcus	Ampicillin 30 mg/kg/day IV, IM or 50 mg/kg/day PO div q8h x 10 days	If culture remains positive, add an aminoglycoside for synergistic effect

* See pages 16-17 for dosage

14

B. USE OF ANTIMICROBIALS DURING PREGNANCY OR BREAST FEEDING

A number of factors determine the degree of transfer of antibiotics across the placenta: lipid solubility, degree of ionization, molecular weight, protein binding, placental maturation, and placental and fetal blood flow. During the latter part of pregnancy maternal serum concentrations of most antibiotics decrease because of the increased volume of distribution. Fetal serum concentrations of the following drugs are equal to, or only slightly less than, those in the mother: penicillin G, amoxicillin, ampicillin, carbenicillin, methicillin, sulfonamides, trimethoprim, tetracyclines, nitrofurantoin and chloramphenicol. The aminoglycoside concentrations in fetal serum are from 20% to 50% of those in maternal serum. Cephalosporins, nafcillin, oxacillin, clindamycin and colistimethate penetrate poorly (10-15%) and fetal concentrations of erythromycin and dicloxacillin are less than 10% of those in the mother.

Some drugs can cause harm to the pregnant woman or fetus. Drugs that are contraindicated are: ribavirin, amantadine, cinoxacin, ciprofloxacin, norfloxacin, erythromycin estolate, griseofulvin, nalidixic acid, tetracyclines, emetine, lindane and primaquine. Drugs that are considered safe are: penicillins, aztreonam, cephalosporins, erythromycin base, methenamine mandelate, spectinomycin, nystatin, chloroquine, niclosamide, paromomycin, permethrin, praziquantel, pyrantel pamoate and pyrethrins. Drugs not listed should be used with caution for firm clinical indications. (**The Medical Letter** 29:61, 1987).

Concentrations of antibiotics in human breast milk are not well studied. Isoniazid, metronidazole, trimethoprim and sulfonamides occur in equal concentrations in maternal serum and milk. Tetracyclines, chloramphenicol and erythromycin are found in breast milk in concentrations 50% to 75% of those in serum. Breast milk concentrations of penicillin G and V, aminoglycosides, nalidixic acid, oxacillin, novobiocin, various cephalosporins, and nitrofurantoin have been reported to be less than 25% of the maternal serum concentrations. Because these are microgram amounts they would not be ingested by the infant in therapeutic amounts.

For example, if an infant took 110 cc/kg body weight of breast milk containing 10 mcg/ml isoniazid in a day, this would amount to a "dose" of 1.1 mg/kg/day. The same infant ingesting milk containing 10 mg/dl of sulfonamide would receive 11 mg/kg/day. On the other hand, with a penicillin V concentration of 0.1 mcg/ml in breast milk the amount of penicillin taken in by the infant would be only 0.011 mg/kg/day.

The AAP Committee on Drugs recommends that breast feeding be discontinued 12-24 hours before treating a nursing mother with metronidazole. Other antibiotics are usually compatible with breast feeding but they warn about the possibility of inducing hemolysis in babies with G-6-PD deficiency by nalidixic acid, nitrofurantoin or sulfa drugs. (Transfer of Drugs and Other Chemicals into Human Milk. **Pediatrics** 1989;84:924)

NEWBORN

15

C. TABLE OF ANTIBIOTIC DOSAGES FOR NEONATES

Antibiotics	Routes	Weight ≤1200g Age 0-4 wk	Weight 1200-2000g Age 0-7 days	Weight 1200-2000g >7 days	Weight > 2000g Age 0-7 days	Weight > 2000g >7 days
			Dosages (mg/kg) and Intervals of Administration			
Amikacin	IV, IM	7.5 q12h	7.5 q12h	7 q8h	10 q12h	30 q8h
Ampicillin, Meningitis	IV, IM	50 q12h	50 q12h	50 q8h	50 q8h	50 q6h
Other diseases		25 q12h	25 q12h	25 q8h	25 q8h	25 q6h
Aztreonam	IV, IM	30 q12h	30 q12h	30 q8h	30 q8h	30 q6h
Cefazolin	IV, IM	20 q12h	20 q12h	20 q12h	20 q12h	20 q8h
Cefotaxime	IV, IM	50 q12h	50 q12h	50 q8h	50 q12h	50 q8h
Ceftazidime	IV, IM	50 q12h	50 q12h	50 q8h	30 q8h	50 q8h
Ceftriaxone	IV, IM	50 q24h	50 q24h	50 q24h	50 q24h	75 q24h
Cephalothin	IV	20 q12h	20 q12h	20 q8h	20 q8h	20 q6h
Chloramphenicol	IV, PO	22 q24h	25 q24h	25 q24h	25 q24h	25 q12h
Clindamycin	IV, IM, PO	5 q12h	5 q12h	5 q8h	5 q8h	5 q6h
Erythromycin	PO	10 q12h	10 q12h	10 q8h	10 q12h	10 q8h
Gentamicin	IV, IM	2.5 q18-24h	2.5 q12h	2.5 q8h	2.5 q12h	2.5 q8h
Kanamycin	IV, IM	7.5 q12h	7.5 q12h	7 q8h	10 q12h	10 q8h

16

Drug	Route					
Methicillin Meningitis	IV, IM	50 q12h	50 q12h	50 q8h	50 q8h	50 q6h
Other diseases		25 q12h	25 q12h	25 q8h	25 q8h	25 q6h
Metronidazole	IV, PO	7.5 q48h	7.5 q24h	7.5 q12h	7.5 q12h	15 q12h
Mezlocillin	IV, IM	75 q12h	75 q12h	75 q8h	75 q12h	75 q8h
Oxacillin	IV, IM	25 q12h	25 q12h	30 q8h	25 q8h	37.5 q6h
Nafcillin	IV	25 q12h	25 q12h	25 q8h	20 q8h	37.5 q6h
Netilmicin	IV, IM	2.5 q18-24h	2.5 q12h	2.5 q8h	2.5 q12h	2.5 q8h
Penicillin G Meningitis	IV	50,000 U q12h	50,000 U q12h	75,000 U q8h	50,000 U q8h	50,000 U q6h
Other diseases		25,000 U q12h	25,000 U q12h	25,000 U q8h	20,000 U q8h	25,000 U q6h
Penicillin G Benzathine	IM		50,000 U (one dose)	50,000 U (one dose)	50,000 U (one dose)	50,000 U (one dose)
Procaine			50,000 U q24h	50,000 U q24h	50,000 U q24h	50,000 U q24
Ticarcillin	IV, IM	75 q12h	75 q12h	75 q8h	75 q8h	75 q6h
Tobramycin	IV, IM	2.5 q18-24h	2 q12h	2 q8h	2 q12h	2 q8h
Vancomycin	IV	15 q24h	10 q12h	10 q8h	15 q12h	10 q8h

Recommendations for infants weighing <1000g based on Prober et al, **Pediatr Infect Dis J** 1990;9:111

VI. ANTIMICROBIAL THERAPY ACCORDING TO CLINICAL SYNDROMES

NOTES:

1. This tabulation should be considered a rough guideline for the "average" patient. Deviations should be made according to physiologic peculiarities of the patient. Dosages recommended are for patients with normal or nearly normal hydration, renal function and hepatic function. See Section XII for patients with impaired renal function and Section XV for dosages based on square meters of body surface area.

2. Duration of treatment should be individualized. The periods recommended are based on common practice and general experience. Critical evaluations of duration of therapy have been carried out in very few diseases.

3. Diseases are arranged by body systems. Consult the index for the alphabetized listing of diseases and Section VII for the alphabetized listing of etiologic agents and for uncommon agents not included in this Section.

Clinical Diagnosis	Therapy	Comments
A. SKIN AND SOFT TISSUE INFECTIONS		
Streptococcal cellulitis (erysipelas)	Penicillin G 50,000-100,000 u/kg/day, IV div q4-6h initially; then penicillin V 50 mg (80,000 u)/kg/day PO div q6-8h x 10 days	NOTE: Erythromycin for penicillin-allergic patients These dosages may be un-necessarily large but little clinical experience with smaller dosages
Lymphangitis, lympha-denitis, blistering dactylitis (streptococcal)	Penicillin V 25-50 mg (40,000-80,000 u)/kg/day PO div q6-8h OR erythromycin 40-50 mg/kg/day PO div q8-12h; x 10 days	For severe disease, penicillin IV (as above)
Impetigo	Mupirocin topically to lesions t.i.d.; OR (for extensive lesions) erythromycin (as above) or cefadroxil 30 mg/kg/day PO div q12h	Bathe daily; often mixed streptococcal and staphylococcal infection
Bullous impetigo, staphylococcal scarlet fever	Cefadroxil 30 mg/kg/day PO div q12h OR cloxacillin 50 mg/kg/day PO div q6h x 5-7 days	Other anti-staphylococcal drugs can be used

18

Condition	Treatment	Notes
Scalded skin syndrome	Nafcillin (or related drug) 150 mg/kg/day IV div q6h initially; then cloxacillin OR cefadroxil OR cephradine/cephalexin (as above) x 5-7 days	Burow's or Zephiran compresses for intertrigenous areas
Pyoderma, abscesses, cervical adenitis, Ludwig's angina (streptococcal, staphylococcal)	Cefadroxil OR cloxacillin OR cephradine/cephalexin (as above); x5-10 days	I & D when indicated; Nafcillin IV for serious infections
Necrotizing fasciitis (streptococcal, staphylococcal)	Nafcillin 150 mg/kg/day IV div q6h x 10 days (add aminoglycoside or ceftazidime if Gram-negative infection suspected)	Debridement; Watch for hypocalcemia, hypoproteinemia; Occasionally due to Gram-negative organisms
Buccal cellulitis (*Haemophilus*) or cellulitis of unknown etiology	Cefuroxime 100-150 mg/kg/day IV, IM div q8h OR chloramphenicol 50-75 mg/kg/day IV, PO div q6h; Alternatives: cefotaxime 100-150 mg/kg/day IV div q6h OR ceftriaxone 50 mg/kg IM, IV once daily; x 5-7 days	R/O meningitis; LARGER DOSAGES NEEDED FOR MENINGITIS
Suppurative myositis (Staphylococcal) (Syn: tropical myositis, pyomyositis)	Nafcillin 150 mg/kg/day IV div q6h x 7-10 days Alternatives: other anti-staphylococcal beta-lactams, vancomycin	Surgical drainage or excision when needed
Gas gangrene (clostridial)	Penicillin G 250,000 u/kg/day IV div q4h x 10 days; Consider hyperbaric oxygen therapy	Antitoxin was of doubtful efficacy and is no longer available
Non-tuberculous (atypical) mycobacterial adenitis	Total surgical excision is usually curative and antimicrobial therapy is not necessary.	If surgical excision not possible, rifampin therapy or other drugs based on susceptibility tests
Tuberculous adenitis	As for pulmonary tuberculosis (See page 26)	Surgical excision usually not indicated

19

Clinical Diagnosis	Therapy	Comments
Animal and human bites	Augmentin 20-40 mg/kg/day PO div q8h x 5-7 days	Human bites often mixed aerobes and anaerobes; Consider rabies prophylaxis for animal bites; Tetanus prophylaxis
		SEE SECTION IV FOR DISCUSSION OF ORAL ANTIBIOTIC THERAPY
B. SKELETAL INFECTIONS		
Suppurative arthritis		Needle aspiration or surgical open drainage; Physiotherapy
- Newborns	See Section V	
- Infants (*Haemophilus*, streptococci, *Staphylococcus*	Cefuroxime 100-150 mg/kg/day IV, IM div q8h OR (for streptococcus) penicillin G 100,000 u/kg/day IV div q4-6h x 14 days or longer OR (for *Staphylococcus*) nafcillin 150 mg/kg/day IV div q6h; x 21 days or longer	Perform LP in patients with *Haemophilus*; LARGER DOSAGES NEEDED FOR MENINGITIS
- Children (*Staphylococcus*, streptococci)	Nafcillin 150 mg/kg/day IV div q6h x 3 weeks or longer; Alternatives: other beta-lactams, clindamycin; vancomycin for methicillin-resistant staphylococci	Change to penicillin G if streptococcus or susceptible pneumococcus
- Gonococcal arthritis or tenosynovitis	Ceftriaxone 25-50 mg/kg once daily IV, IM OR (if susceptible) penicillin G 100,000 u/kg/day IV div q6h x 7-10 days	3-5 days therapy adequate in adults, but not tested in children
- Other bacteria	See Section VII for preferred antibiotics	

Osteomyelitis or osteochondritis

- Newborn

See Section V

Surgery; Immobilization

- Acute, initial therapy (usually _Staphyloccocus_, streptococci, _Haemophilus_)

Infants: cefuroxime 100-150 mg/kg/day IV, IM div q8h; Children > 4 yrs: nafcillin 150 mg/kg/day IV, div q6h x 3 weeks or longer. Alternatives: other beta-lactams, clindamycin

In children add cefotaxime to nafcillin if Gram-negative rods in pus, pending culture and susceptibility results

- Acute, other organisms

See Section VII for preferred antibiotics

- _Pseudomonas aeruginosa_

Ceftazidime 150 mg/kg/day IV, IM div q8h OR mezlocillin or ticarcillin 200-300 mg/kg/day IV div q6h AND (compromised host) gentamicin 5 mg/kg/day IM, IV or amikacin 15-20 mg/kg/day IM, IV div q8h; x 10 days

7-10 days therapy adequate in normal host providing that complete surgical debridement done

- Chronic (staphylococcal)

Dicloxacillin 75-100 mg/kg/day PO div q6h OR cephradine/cephalexin 100-150 mg/kg/day PO div q6h; x 6-12 months

Surgery; Monitor serum for bactericidal titer (See Section IV for details)

C. EYE INFECTIONS

Hordeolum (sty) or chalazion

None (Topical antibiotic not necessary)

Warm compresses; I & D when necessary

Acute conjunctivitis

Polymyxin B-bacitracin or sulfacetamid ophthalmic crops q2h or ointment q4-6h

See page 9 for chlamydial, gonococcal, pseudomonas infection

Herpetic conjunctivitis

Trifluoridine sol'n 1 drop q2-3h while awake x 7-14 days; OR vidarabine ointment topically q3h until 1 week after healing

Consider steroids if keratitis present (refer to ophthalmologist)

21

Clinical Diagnosis	Therapy	Comments
Periorbital cellulitis (Pre-septal infection)		
- Associated with sinusitis	Cefuroxime 100-150 mg/kg/day IV, IM div q8h x 5-7 days	Follow with oral antibiotic (See page 24)
- Idiopathic (*Haemophilus* or pneumococcal)	Cefuroxime 100-150 mg/kg/day IV, IM div q8h <u>OR</u> chloramphenicol 50-75 mg/kg/day IV, PO div q6h; x 7-10 days	Lumbar puncture to R/O meningitis; LARGER DOSAGES NEEDED FOR MENINGITIS
- Associated with periorbital skin lesion (streptococcal, staphylococcal)	Nafcillin 150 mg/kg/day IV div q6h x 7-10 days	Oral antistaphylococcal antibiotic for less severe infection
Orbital cellulitis (Post-septal infection)	Nafcillin 150 mg/kg/day IV div q6h <u>AND</u> chloramphenicol 75-100 mg/kg/day IV, PO div q6h x 10-14 days	Usually staphylococcal or Gram-negative bacilli; Surgical drainage of pus
Dacryocystitis	No antibiotic usually; when needed, based on Gram stain and culture of pus	Warm compresses; May require surgical probing of naso-lachrymal duct
Endophthalmitis		NOTE: Subconjunctival/sub-tenon antibiotic often needed; steroids commonly used
- Staphylococcal	Nafcillin 150 mg/kg/day IV div q6h x 10-14 days; Alternatives: other beta-lactams or vancomycin	Penicillin for susceptible organisms
- Pneumococcal, meningococcal	Penicillin G 250,000 u/kg/day IV div q4h x 10-14 days (chloramphenicol or vancomycin for penicillin-insensitive pneumococci)	R/O meningitis

22

- Gonococcal

Ceftriaxone 50 mg/kg once daily IV, IM x 7 days or longer

- *Pseudomonas*

Mezlocillin or ticarcillin 200-300 mg/kg/day IV div q4-6h AND gentamicin 6 mg/kg/day IM, or amikacin 15-20 mg/kg/day IM, IV div q6h x 10-14 days

Piperacillin or ceftazidime are alternatives

Retinitis

- Cytomegalovirus

Ganciclovir (for dosage see Section X)

D. EAR AND SINUS INFECTIONS

External otitis, bacterial

Optimal therapy unknown; cleaning canal of detritus important; antibiotic or antibiotic-steroid drops (e.g. Cortisporin suspension) customarily used but efficacy not proved

Wick moistened with Burow's sol'n used for marked swelling of canal; For "swimmer's ear", VoSol or alcohol-vinegar mixture to canal after water exposure

External otitis, fungal (otomycosis)

Topical 1/2 alcohol - 1/2 vinegar sol'n OR 25% M-cresyl acetate (Cresylate) t.i.d.

Usually *Aspergillus*; Debride canal

Furuncle of external canal

Cefadroxil 30 mg/kg/day div q12h OR cloxacillin 50 mg/kg/day div q6-8h OR cephradine/cephalexin 50 mg/kg/day div q6-8h

I & D; Antibiotic not necessary unless cellulitis

Bullous myringitis

Antibiotics, as for otitis media with effusion (see below)

Current concept is that this is simply one manifestation of acute otitis media

23

Clinical Diagnosis	Therapy	Comments
Otitis media, acute with effusion		
- Newborns	See Section V	
- Infants and children (pneumococcus, *Haemophilus*, *Moraxella* most common)	Amoxicillin or Augmentin 40 mg/kg/day PO div q8h; OR erythromycin-sulfa combination 40 mg/kg/day of erythro component PO div q6h OR cefaclor 40 mg/kg/day PO div q8-12h OR TMP/SMX 6-8 mg/kg/day of TMP component PO div q12h OR cefixime 8 mg/kg once daily or div q12h; x 5-10 days	Gram stain and culture of pus if spontaneous rupture; IF prior antibiotic therapy or compromised host, suspect unusual infection and do tympanocentesis for culture

A Note on Acute Otitis Media with Effusion: There are several effective antibiotic regimens for management of OME. Customarily amoxicillin is used initially and other drugs are given for amoxicillin failures or relapses. The physician should consider advantages and disadvantages regarding antibacterial spectrum, palatability of suspensions, and cost. TMP/SMX is not effective for Group A streptococcal infection. When prophylaxis is indicated, use amoxicillin or sulfa drug in one-half the therapeutic dose once or twice daily.

Mastoiditis, acute (pneumococcus, staphylococcus, Gr. A streptococcus; *Haemophilus* rare)	Nafcillin 150 mg/kg/day IV div q6h OR cefuroxime 100-150 mg/kg/day IV, IM div q8h x 10 days; Alternatives: other beta-lactams or vancomycin	R/O meningitis; Surgery as needed; Change to oral therapy after clinical improvement
Mastoiditis, chronic	Antibiotics only for acute superinfections (according to culture of drainage); also, when chronic *Pseudomonas* infection, mezlocillin or ticarcillin 200-300 mg/kg/day IV div q4-6h x 5-7 days	Daily cleansing of ear important; After resolution, use amoxicillin or sulfa prophylaxis for otitis; If no response, surgery
Sinusitis, acute (*Haemophilus*, pneumococcus, streptococcus, *Moraxella*)	Same as for acute otitis media but 14-21 days may be needed	Sinus irrigations when indicated

E. NOSE AND THROAT INFECTIONS

Diphtheria

Penicillin G 150,000 u/kg/day IV div q6h OR erythromycin 50 mg/kg/day PO x 7-10 days

Plus antitoxin; Isolation until 3 daily nose and throat cultures negative

Streptococcal tonsilopharyngitis, scarlet fever and peritonsillar cellulitis

Penicillin V 25-50 mg/kg/day PO div q6-8h x 10 days OR benzathine penicillin 25,000 u/kg IM (max 1.2 million u) as a single dose; Alternatives: oral cephalosporins

Erythromycin or clindamycin for penicillin-allergic patients (Caution: 5% of Group A strep resistant)

Epiglottitis (Aryepiglottitis, Supraglottitis)

Cefuroxime 100-150 mg/kg/day IV, IM div q8h OR chloramphenicol 50-75 mg/kg/day IV div q6h x 5-7 days; Alternatives: cefotaxime, ceftriaxone

Provide airway; Almost always caused by *Haemophilus influenzae*, type b

Retropharyngeal or lateral pharyngeal cellulitis or abscess

Clindamycin 30 mg/kg/day PO, IV, IM div q6h OR nafcillin 150 mg/kg/day IV div q6h and chloramphenicol 50-75 mg/kg/day IV,PO

Usually aerobes and anaerobes; I & D when pus present; Consider tonsillectomy for peritonsillar abscess

F. LOWER RESPIRATORY INFECTIONS

Respiratory syncytial virus infection (bronchiolitis, pneumonia)

Ribavirin 6g vial (20 mg/ml in sterile water) aerosolized by SPAG-2 over 18-20 hr period daily x 3-5 days

Treat only for severe disease or patients with underlying cardiopulmonary disease

Pertussis

Erythromycin (estolate preferred) 50 mg/kg/day PO div q6h x 10 days (re-administer vomited doses, or change to ampicillin 100 mg/kg/day IV, IM div q6h)

Hospitalize young babies; Avoid mist therapy; Avoid cough suppressants; Isolate until 2 daily cultures negative or for 10 days

25

Clinical Diagnosis	Therapy	Comments
Tuberculosis		
- Primary	Isoniazid 10-15 mg/kg/day (max 300 mg) PO div q12-24h AND rifampin 10-15 mg/kg/day (max 600 mg) PO, IV div q24h; OR: isoniazid AND ethambutol 15 mg/kg/day div q24h; x 9 months	With ethambutol, monitor for optic nerve toxicity; Observe for clinical signs of hepatic toxicity
	Alternative regimen #1: Isoniazid and rifampin (as above) x 1 month; FOLLOWED BY: isoniazid 20-40 mg/kg (max 900 mg) AND rifampin 10-20 mg/kg (max 600 mg) twice weekly x 8 months	Arkansas regimen (**Pediatrics** 72:801, 1983)
	Alternative regimen #2: Isoniazid and rifampin (as above) daily for 6 months with pyrizinamide 25-30 mg/kg/day PO div q8h for first 2 months	
- Skin test conversion	Isoniazid 10-15 mg/kg/day (max 300 mg) PO daily x 9 months	Single drug Rx if no clinical or radiographic evidence of disease
- Exposed infant < 6 yrs, or immunocompromised patient	Isoniazid 10-15 mg/kg PO daily x 3 mos after last exposure	If PPD remains negative, and child well, stop prophylaxis
Lung abscess		
- Primary, putrid (i.e., foul-smelling)	Clindamycin 30 mg/kg/day PO, IM, IV div q6-8h; OR penicillin G 100,000 u/kg/day IV div q4-6h AND chloramphenicol 50-75 mg/kg/day IV, PO div q6h; x 10 days or longer	Polymicrobial infection with aerobes and anaerobes

- Primary, non-putrid	Cefuroxime 100-150 mg/kg/day IV, IM div q8h or other beta-lactamase-resistant beta-lactam; x 10 days or longer	Bronchoscopy necessary if abscess fails to drain; Surgical excision rarely necessary
- Secondary to other focus of infection (osteomyelitis, etc.)	Nafcillin 150 mg/kg/day IV div q6h x 10 days or longer OR other beta-lactams	Usually staphylococcal; cephalosporin for coliforms
Pneumonia in immunosuppressed, neutropenic host	Nafcillin 150 mg/kg/day IV div q6h or vancomycin 40 mg/kg/day IV div q6h (if methicillin-resistant Staph suspected) AND ceftazidime 150 mg/kg/day IV div q8h; Alternative: mezlocillin or ticarcillin 200-300 mg/kg/day IV div q6h AND amikacin 15-22.5 mg/kg/day or gentamicin 6 mg/kg/day IM, IV div q8h AND nafcillin (as above)	Consider opportunist bacteria, pneumocystis, cytomegalovirus, fungi, tuberculosis; biopsy of lung may be needed to establish diagnosis
Acute pulmonary exacerbations of cystic fibrosis	Ticarcillin 300-400 mg/kg/day IV div q4h AND tobramycin 6-10 mg/kg/day IM, IV div q6-8h; Alternatives: other anti-*Pseudomonas* beta-lactams and aminoglycosides OR ceftazidime 150 mg/kg/day IV div q8h; x 7-10 days OR aztreonam 200 mg/kg/day IV div q6h	Larger than normal dosages required in most patients with cystic fibrosis; Monitor peak serum concentrations of aminoglycosides
Pneumocystis carinii **pneumonia**	(See page 56)	
Bronchitis, acute	No antibiotic for most cases (viral); if bacterial infection suspected, use same drugs as for acute otitis or sinusitis (page 24)	*Haemophilus, Branhamella,* pneumococcus most common pathogens in adults and (?) in children
Allergic bronchopulmonary aspergillosis	Prednisone 0.5 mg/kg every other day	Larger dosages may lead to tissue invasion

Clinical Diagnosis	Therapy	Comments
Pneumonia with empyema		Initial therapy based on Gram stain of empyema fluid
- Pneumococcal, Group A streptococcal	Penicillin G 150,000 u/kg/day IV div q4-6h x 10 days (Change to PO penicillin V in same dosage after clinical improvement); Alternatives: cephalosporins, clindamycin	Closed chest tube drainage of purulent fluid
- Staphylococcal	Nafcillin 150 mg/kg/day IV div q6h OR vancomycin 40 mg/kg/day div q6h x 21 days or longer (Alternatives: cephalosporins)	Closed chest tube drainage of empyema
- *Haemophilus influenzae* b or pneumonia of unestablished etiology (< 5 yrs of age)	Cefuroxime 100-150 mg/kg/day IV, IM div q8h; OR ampicillin 150 mg/kg/day IV, IM div q6h AND chloramphenicol 50-75 mg/kg/day IV, PO div q6h x 10-14 days; Alternatives: cefotaxime 100-150 mg/kg/day IV div q6h or ceftriaxone 50 mg/kg IV, IM once daily	Closed chest tube drainage; R/O meningitis; LARGER DOSAGES NEEDED FOR MENINGITIS
Lobar or segmental consolidation		
- *Haemophilus*, or unknown etiology	Cefuroxime 100-150 mg/kg/day IV, IM div q8h x 10 days	Change to PO cefaclor after improvement
- Pneumococcal	Penicillin G 150,000 u/kg/day IV div q4-6h x 10 days. Alternatives: cephalosporins	Change to PO penicillin V in same dosage after improvement
- *Klebsiella pneumoniae*	Gentamicin 6 mg/kg/day IM, IV div q8h x 10 days or longer OR amikacin 15-20 mg/kg/day IM div q8h; (Alternative: cefotaxime 150 mg/kg/day IV, IM div q6h)	Suspect if distended lobe; Abscesses common but empyema rare

Bronchopneumonia

- Mild to moderate illness

No antibiotic therapy unless epidemiological/clinical reasons to suspect specific pathogen other than virus

Most viral; Broad spectrum antibiotics increase risk of superinfection

- Serious, life-threatening illness

Initially, until etiology established, nafcillin 150 mg/kg/day IV div q6h AND gentamicin 6 mg/kg/day or amikacin 15-22.5 mg/kg/day IM, IV div q8h (Cefotaxime or cefuroxime may be effective)

Consider needle aspiration of lung to establish diagnosis (Gram stain and culture of aspirate); Tracheal aspirate Gram stain culture may be helpful

Afebrile pneumonia syndrome of early infancy

Supportive, or (if chlamydia suspected) erythromycin 40 mg/kg/day PO div q6h x 14 days

Most viral or chlamydial; often interstitial infiltrate

Other pneumonias of established etiology

29

- *Chlamydia pneumoniae* (TWAR), *C. psittaci* or *C. trachomatis*

Erythromycin OR tetracycline (pts >7 yrs) (Ampicillin for *C. trachomatis*)

For dosage see Section X

- Cytomegalovirus

Ganciclovir

For dosage see Section X

- *E. coli, Enterobacter* spp.

An aminoglycoside or cephalosporin

For dosage see Section X

- *Francisella tularensis*

Gentamicin or streptomycin

See page 42

- Fungi

Amphotericin B or combined therapy

For dosage see Section VIII

- Influenza A

Amantadine

For dosage, see page 40

(continued on next page)

Clinical Diagnosis	Therapy	Comments
Other pneumonias of established etiology (cont.)		
- Legionnaire's Disease	Erythromycin and (?) rifampin	For dosage, see Section X
- Melioidosis	See page 41	
- *Mycoplasma pneumoniae*	Erythromycin or tetracycline	For dosage, see Section X
- *Paragonimus westermani*	Praziquantel	For dosage, see page 61
- *Pseudomonas aeruginosa*	Anti-*Pseudomonas* penicillin <u>AND</u> amino-glycoside; <u>OR</u> ceftazidime	For dosage, see Section X
G. HEART INFECTIONS		
Purulent pericarditis		SURGICAL DRAINAGE OF PUS
- *Staphylococcus aureus*	Nafcillin 150 mg/kg/day IV div q6h <u>OR</u> (for methicillin-resistant staphylococci) vancomycin 40 mg/kg/day IV div q6h x 3 wks or longer	Change to penicillin G if susceptible
- *Haemophilus influenzae* b	Cefuroxime 100-150 mg/kg/day IV, IM div q8h x 10-14 days; Alternatives: cefotaxime, ceftriaxone	Ampicillin for beta-lactamase-negative strains
- Pneumococcus, meningococcus, Group A streptococcus	Penicillin G 150,000 u/kg/day IV, IM div q4-6h x 10-14 days	Vancomycin for penicillin-insensitive pneumococci
- Coliform bacilli	Cefotaxime 100-150 mg/kg/day IV, IM div q6-8h x 3 wks or longer; Alternatives: other cephalosporins, aminoglycoside	Alternative drugs depending on susceptibilities
- Tuberculous	(See page 26)	Corticosteroids for first 2-3 months

30

Endocarditis

- Viridans streptococcus

Penicillin G 150,000 u/kg/day IV div q4-6h x 30 days (optional: AND streptomycin 30 mg/kg/day IM div q12h during first 14 days); OR vancomycin 40 mg/kg/day IV div q6h

Monitor serum bactericidal activity; See Section IV for discussion of oral therapy

- Enterococcus

Ampicillin 150 mg/kg/day IV, IM div q6h x 30 days AND gentamicin 6 mg/kg/day IM, IV div q8h OR penicillin G 250,000 u/kg/day IV div q4-6h AND streptomycin 30 mg/kg/day IM div q12h; x 30 days

Longest experience with the penicillin-streptomycin regimen; Combined Rx used for synergistic bactericidal activity

- *Staphylococcus aureus,*
  Staphylococcus epidermidis

Nafcillin 150 mg/kg/day IV div q6h x 6 wks OR, for methicillin-resistant staphylococci, vancomycin 40 mg/kg/day IV div q6h; Consider adding rifampin or aminoglycoside for synergistic effect

Surgery may be necessary in acute phase; Avoid cephalo-sporins because of conflicting data on efficacy

- Pneumococcus, gonococcus, Group A streptococcus

Penicillin G 150,000 u/kg/day IV div q4-6h x 14 days (vancomycin for penicillin-insensitive pneumococci)

Ceftriaxone for gonococcus until susceptibilities known

- Prophylaxis for:

If penicillin allergy:

- Dental and upper respiratory procedures

Amoxicillin PO 50 mg/kg 1 hr before procedure and 25 mg/kg 6 hr later
OR
Ampicillin IM, IV 50 mg/kg 30 min before AND gentamicin IM, IV 2 mg/kg 30 min before

Erythromycin 20 mg/kg 2 hr before and 10 mg/kg 6 hr later

Vancomycin IV 20 mg/kg during 1 hr before

- Genitourinary and gastrointestinal procedures

Amoxicillin PO (as above) OR ampicillin IM, IV AND gentamicin IM, IV (as above)

Vancomycin IV (as above) AND gentamicin IM, IV (as above)

Clinical Diagnosis	Therapy	Comments
H. GASTROINTESTINAL INFECTIONS	(See Section IX for parasitic infections)	
Shigellosis	Trimethoprim/sulfamethoxazole 10 mg TMP-50 mg SMX/kg/day PO, IV div q12h x 5 days OR (for susceptible strains) ampicillin 100 mg/kg/day IV, IM, PO div q6h	Tetracycline, chloramphenicol, absorbable sulfas, nalidixic acid also effective when *Shigella* susceptible; Avoid anti-peristaltic drugs
Salmonellosis	None for usual self-limited diarrhea OR 50 mg/kg/day PO div q6h x 5-7 days OR TMP/SMX as for shigellosis (For typhoid fever see page 42)	Treat infants with bacteremia, compromised hosts and those with septic clinical picture or colitis (IV antibiotics for bacteremia)
Escherichia coli		
- Enteropathogenic	Neomycin 100 mg/kg/day PO div q6-8h OR colistin 15 mg/kg/day PO div q6-8h x 3-5 days	Most traditional "entero-pathogenic" strains not toxigenic or invasive
- Enterotoxigenic	Trimethoprim-sulfamethoxazole (as for shigellosis) OR neomycin or colistin PO	Most illnesses brief and self-limited
- Enteroinvasive	(?) Orally absorbable antibiotic, such as ampicillin, amoxicillin or trimethoprim-sulfamethoxazole	No controlled clinical trials on which to base a recommendation
"Turista" (Traveler's Diarrhea)	As for enterotoxigenic *E. coli* above	50-75% of cases due to toxigenic *E. coli*; If not improved after 5 days, investigate for *Shigella*, *Giardia*, etc.
Yersinia enterocolitica	Antimicrobial therapy not of value	May mimic appendicitis

Campylobacter jejuni	Erythromycin 40 mg/kg/day PO div q6h x 5 days	Abdominal pain may mimic acute surgical abdomen
Aeromonas sp.	(?) Trimethoprim-sulfamethoxazole as for shigellosis	Efficacy not established
Antibiotic-associated colitis	Vancomycin 50 mg/kg/day PO div q6h x 7 days; Alternatives: metronidazole 20 mg/kg/day PO div q6h; bacitracin 2000 u/kg/day PO div q6h	Due to overgrowth of Cl. difficile in gut; vancomycin IV may be less effective than PO
Perirectal abscess	Clindamycin 30-40 mg/kg/day IV, PO div q5-8h AND aminoglycoside or cephalosporin	*S. aureus* common but may be mixed with coliforms, anaerobes; Surgical drainage

I. GENITOURINARY AND SEXUALLY TRANSMITTED INFECTIONS

		CONSIDERATION OF TESTING FOR HIV INFECTION IN CHILDREN WITH SEXUALLY TRANSMITTED DISEASES
Genital herpes infection	Acyclovir one-200 mg cap PO 5 x daily x 7-10 days OR (for severe disease) acyclovir 15 mg/kg/day as 1 hr IV infusion div q8h x 5-7 days	Most effective when started early in course of infection; Does not prevent recurrence; Topical therapy less effective
Urinary tract infection		
- Acute cystitis	Trisulfapyrimidines or sulfisoxazole 120-150 mg/kg/day PO div q6h OR amoxicillin 30 mg/kg/day div q6-8h x 7-10 days; For recurrent infections, trimethoprim-sulfamethoxazole 6 mg TMP-30 mg SMX/kg/day div q12h	"In vivo" susceptibility test: follow-up culture after 36-48 hrs treatment. If culture positive, change treatment according to *in vitro* susceptibilities

33

Clinical Diagnosis	Therapy	Comments
Urinary tract infection (cont.)		
- Acute pyelonephritis	Gentamicin 6 mg/kg/day IV, IM div q8h OR trimethoprim-sulfamethoxazole 6 mg TMP-30 mg SMX/kg/day PO, IV div q12h x 10 days	Parenteral drug if sepsis suspected; Change to appropriate oral drug after clinical response
- Prophylaxis for recurrent bacteriuria	Trimethoprim-sulfamethoxazole 2 mg TMP-10 mg SMX/kg PO q1-2 days OR nitrofurantoin 1-2 mg/kg PO q1-2 days at bedtime	Prophylaxis for patients with grade 3 or 4 reflux or frequent infections
Epididymitis	(For non-sexually active) nafcillin 150 mg/kg/day IV div q6h AND chloramphenicol 50-75 mg/kg/day IV, PO div q6h; x 7-10 days	Usually due to *Haemophilus* or *S. aureus* in young children; Treat as for gonorrhea and chlamydia in older children
Trichomoniasis	See Section IX	
Vaginitis or cervicitis		
- Vulvovaginal Candidiasis	See Section VIII	
- *Shigella*	As for diarrhea (see page 32)	50% have bloody discharge usually not associated with diarrhea
- Chlamydial	Doxycycline 4 mg/kg/day (max. 200 mg) PO div q12h OR Tetracycline (Pts > 7 yrs) 40 mg/kg/day PO div q6h OR trisulfapyrimidines or sulfisoxazole 120-150 mg/kg/day PO div q6h OR erythromycin 40 mg/kg/day PO div q6h x 7-10 days	*Chlamydia* occurs in pre-pubertal as well as post-pubertal children
- Bacterial vaginosis (formerly nonspecific vaginitis)	Metronidazole 15-20 mg/kg/day PO div q8h x 7-10 days	Caused by synergy of *Gardnerella* with anaerobes

Gonorrhea

Condition	Treatment	Notes
- Newborns	See Section V	Ceftriaxone preferred; Serologic test for syphilis; Repeat in 3 mos. if treated with something other than penicillin; Social evaluation re possibility of child abuse; Follow with treatment for presumed chlamydia
- Genital infections	Treatment regimens of demonstrated efficacy for children: 1) Ceftriaxone 5 mg/kg (max 250 mg) IM as single dose 2) Procaine penicillin G 100,000 u/kg IM as single dose (2 injection sites) AND probenecid 25 mg/kg PO (max 1g) 3) Amoxicillin 50 mg/kg PO as single dose AND probenecid 25 mg/kg PO 4) Spectinomycin 40 mg/kg IM as single dose 5) Cefuroxime 25 mg/kg IM as single dose	
- Disseminated gonococcal infection	Ceftriaxone 1g IM, IV once daily OR cefotaxime 4g/day IV div q8h (adult dosages)	No controlled studies in children; follow treatment recommendations for adults with appropriate dosage modifications

Syphilis

Condition	Treatment	Notes
- Congenital	See Section V	See CDC 1989 <u>Sexually Transmitted Diseases Treatment Guidelines</u>
- Primary, secondary	Benzathine penicillin G 2,400,000 u IM (approximately 50,000 u/kg) in 2 injection sites OR doxycycline 4 mg/kg/day (max 200 mg) PO div q12h x 14 days OR tetracycline 30 g total dosage given 2 g/day in 4 doses for 14 days (approximately 40 mg/kg/day) OR erythromycin (same dosage as tetracycline)	Follow up serologic tests at 3, 6 and 12 months; Do not use benzathine-procaine penicillin mixtures

(continued on next page)

35

Clinical Diagnosis	Therapy	Comments
Syphilis (cont.)		
- Syphilis of more than 1 year duration	Benzathine penicillin G 2,400,000 u IM (50,000 u/kg) in 2 injection sites weekly for 3 doses OR tetracycline or erythromycin 500 mg q.i.d. x 30 days (approximately 40 mg/kg/day) OR doxycycline 4 mg/kg/day (max 200 mg) PO div q12h	Optimal treatment schedule not established
Chancroid	Ceftriaxone 5 mg/kg (max 250 mg) IM as single dose OR trimethoprim-sulfamethoxazole 6 mg TMP-30 mg SMX/kg/day PO div q12h x 7 days	Serologic test for syphilis; Erythromycin also effective
Lymphogranuloma venereum (*Chlamydia trachomatis*)	Doxycycline 4 mg/kg/day (max 200 mg) PO div q12h OR tetracycline (Pts >7 yrs) 40 mg/kg/day PO div q6h x 21 days	Erythromycin and sulfisoxazole probably effective
Pelvic inflammatory disease	Cefoxitin 2 g IV q6h AND doxycycline 100 mg PO bid OR clindamycin 900 mg IV q8h AND gentamicin 1.5 mg IV, IM q8h	(Adult dosages) Both regimens given until clinical improvement and followed by doxycycline for 10-14 days

J. CENTRAL NERVOUS SYSTEM INFECTIONS

Bacterial meningitis

NOTE: Dexamethasone (0.6 mg/kg/day IV div q6h x4 days) as an adjunct to antibiotic therapy decreases hearing deficits and possibly other neurologic sequelae in *Haemophilus* meningitis and possibly other types. The first dose of dexamethasone is preferably given before the first dose of antibiotic.

- Neonatal   See Section V

36

Haemophilus influenzae b	Cefotaxime 200 mg/kg/day IV div q6h OR ceftriaxone EITHER 100 mg/kg/day IV div q12h OR 80 mg/kg IV, IM once daily OR cefuroxime 240 mg/kg/day IV div q8h. Alternative: Ampicillin 200 mg/kg/day IV div q6h AND chloramphenicol 100 mg/kg/day IV div q6h; x 10 days	Delayed sterilization of CSF reported with cefuroxime; Chloramphenicol can be given PO; Rifampin prophylaxis for patient and contacts according to 1988 Red Book recommendations
- Pneumococcus	Penicillin G 250,000 u/kg/day IV div q4h x 10 days; For penicillin-insensitive pneumococci use chloramphenicol 100 mg/kg/day IV, PO div q6h; for penicillin-resistant pneumococci use vancomycin 60 mg/kg/day IV div q6h (cefotaxime, ceftriaxone may be effective)	Approx 5% of pneumococci relatively resistant ("insensitive") to penicillin; Rare strains are resistant to chloramphenicol
- Meningococcus (Including meningococcemia)	Penicillin G 250,000 u/kg/day IV div q4h x 7 days; NOTE: Regimens given for *Haemophilus* are effective for meningococcal infection	Meningococcal prophylaxis: rifampin 10 mg/kg PO q12h x 4 doses; Trisulfapyrimidines 25 mg/kg PO q12h x 4 doses if organism from index case sulfa-susceptible
- Unknown bacterial, 1-3 mos of age	Ampicillin (as above) AND cefotaxime 200 mg/kg/day IV div q6h	Both "neonatal" and "infant" pathogens encountered in this age group
- Unknown bacterial, after 3 mos of age	As for *Haemophilus* (above)	

(continued on next page)

37

Clinical Diagnosis	Therapy	Comments
(Bacterial meningitis - cont.)		
- Tuberculous	Isoniazid 15 mg/kg/day PO, IM div q12-24h AND rifampin 15 mg/kg/day, IV, PO div q12-24h x 12 mos AND streptomycin 30 mg/kg/day IM div q12h for first 4 weeks of therapy (consider adding pyrazinamide 30 mg/kg/day PO q12-24h for first 2 months)	Hyponatremia from inappropriate ADH common; Ventricular drainage may be necessary; Steroids suppress symptoms but probably do not improve prognosis
Shunt infections		
- *S. epidermidis* or *S. aureus*	Vancomycin 60 mg/kg/day IV div q6h OR nafcillin 150 mg/kg/day (?) PLUS an aminoglycoside or rifampin; x 10-14 days	Surgery for shunt revision usually necessary; May be synergy between antibiotics
- Coliform bacilli	Cefotaxime 200 mg/kg/day IV div q6h OR ampicillin 200 mg/kg/day IV div q6h AND gentamicin 6 mg/kg/day or amikacin 15-20 mg/kg/day IV, IM div q8h; x 21 days or longer	Select appropriate drug based on *in vitro* susceptibilities
Brain abscess	Until etiology established nafcillin or vancomycin (as above) AND cefotaxime (as above) AND metronidazole 30 mg/kg/day IV, PO div q8h; x 7-10 days after surgery	Surgery; Anaerobes common; Add anti-*Pseudomonas* drug if secondary to chronic otitis; Follow abscess size with CT scans
Herpes simplex encephalitis	Acyclovir 30 mg/kg/day as 1 hr or longer IV infusion div q8h OR vidarabine 15 mg/kg as 12 hr or longer IV infusion daily x 10 days	Acyclovir probably more effective
Toxoplasma encephalitis	See Section IX	

K. MISCELLANEOUS SYSTEMIC INFECTIONS

Acquired immunodeficiency syndrome

See HIV infection below

Actinomycosis

Penicillin G 250,000 u/kg/day IV div q4h until improved; thereafter penicillin V 100 mg/kg/day PO div q6h x several months

Surgery as indicated; Tetracycline for penicillin-allergic

Brucellosis

Tetracycline 40 mg/kg/day PO, IV div q6h (IV daily dose should not exceed 2 g) if > 7 yrs; TMP 10 mg/kg-SMX 50 mg/kg/day div q12h if <7 yrs; rifampin (15-20 mg/kg/day div q12h) as second drug may decrease relapses; x 21 days or longer

Add gentamicin 5-6 mg/kg/day IV, IM div q6h for the first 5 days

Cat scratch disease

Supportive; aspiration of pus

Gentamicin, cefoxitin or cefotaxime may be effective

Ehrlichiosis

(See Rickettsial infection below)

Febrile neutropenic patient

Nafcillin (or vancomycin if methicillin resistant Staph is suspected) AND anti-Pseudomonas beta-lactam AND aminoglycoside; OR anti-staphylococcal drug AND ceftazidime

If no response in 5-7 days and no bacterial etiology demonstrated, consider empiric antifungal therapy with amphotericin B; Dosages in Section X

Human immunodeficiency virus infection

Zidovidine 720 mg/m^2/day PO div q6h (dideoxyinosine is in clinical trials in children)

Appropriate monitoring for toxicity; IV formulation not commercially available

Infant botulism

No antibiotic or antitoxin; aminoglycosides potertiate effect of toxin; (trivalent antitoxin for foodborne or wound botulism)

ICU supportive therapy; Enemas to remove constipated stool and toxin is controversial

39

Clinical Diagnosis	Therapy	Comments
Influenza A infection	Amantadine 5 mg/kg/day (max. 200 mg) PO div q12h x 7 days; Ribavirin aerosol (as for RSV infection, page 25) may be effective	Treat within 48-72 hrs of onset; Rx especially for high-risk patients
Kawasaki syndrome	No antibiotics; IV gamma globulin (400 mg/kg daily x 4 days); a single large dose (2g/kg) also reported to be beneficial	Aspirin qs to achieve serum conc of 20-30 mg/dl in acute phase; prolonged low dosage (3-5 mg/kg/day) aspirin Rx may decrease risk of coronary artery disease
Leprosy	Dapsone 1 mg/kg PO daily PLUS clofazimine 1 mg/kg PO daily PLUS rifampin 10 mg/kg PO once monthly	Clofazimine necessary because of increased resistance to dapsone
Leptospirosis	Penicillin G 250,000 u/kg/day IV, IM div q4-6h OR tetracycline 40 mg/kg/day PO div q6h; x 7-10 days	
Lyme Disease	Early disease: penicillin V 50 mg/kg/day PO div q8h OR penicillin G 100,000 u/kg/day IV div q4h OR tetracycline 40-50 mg/kg/day PO div q6h; x 10-14 days	Late disease: penicillin G 250,000 u/kg/day IV div q4h OR ceftriaxone 100 (CNS) or 50 (others) mg/kg once daily IM, IV; x 14 days
Measles	Supportive therapy; ribavirin has been used 15 mg/kg/day IV div q8h x 10 days (double dose on 1st day); Vitamin A therapy reported to be beneficial	Consider ribavirin in severe disease/compromised host; IV formulation not commercially available

40

Melioidosis	<u>Acute sepsis</u>: Ceftazidime 120 mg/kg/day IV div q8h <u>OR</u> chloramphenicol 50-75 mg/kg/day IV, PO div q6h <u>AND</u> trisulfa-pyrimidines or sulfisoxazole 120-150 mg PO div q6h <u>AND</u> an aminoglycoside; x 10-14 days <u>Chronic infection</u>: Trimethoprim-sulfa-methoxazole 8 mg TMP/kg-40 mg SMX/kg/day x several weeks	Ceftazidime more effective than conventional 3 drug therapy in one study Tetracycline for children over 7 years of age
Nocardiosis	Trisulfapyrimidines or sulfisoxazole 120-150 mg/kg/day PO div q6h x 6 weeks or longer; For severe infection, amikacin 15-20 mg/kg/day IM, IV div q8h	Surgery when indicated; Tri-methoprim-sulfamethoxazole or cycloserine as alternatives
Peritonitis		
- Primary	Penicillin G 150,000 u/kg/day IV, IM div q4h x 7-10 days	Usually pneumococcal; Other antibiotics according to culture and susceptibility tests
- Secondary to bowel perforation or appendicitis	Clindamycin 30 mg/kg/day IV, IM div q6h <u>AND</u> gentamicin 6 mg/kg/day IV, IM div q8h x 10 days or longer	Many other regimens claimed to be effective; add ampicillin for enterococcus
- Secondary to peritoneal dialysis	Antibiotic added to dialysate in concen-trations approximating those attained in serum for systemic disease (e.g. 8 mcg/ml for gentamicin; 50 mcg/ml for vancomycin, etc.)	Selection of antibiotic based on organism isolated from peritoneal fluid; Systemic antibiotics if there is accompanying bacteremia
Rickettsial infection	Tetracycline (Pts > 7 yrs) 40 mg/kg/day PO div q6h (Initially can be given IV) <u>OR</u> chloramphenicol 50-75 mg/kg/day IV, PO div q6h; x 10-14 days	Chloramphenicol is preferred for young children

41

Clinical Diagnosis	Therapy	Comments
Tetanus	Penicillin G 100,000 u/kg/day IV div q4-6h x 10 days	Plus antitoxin and sedation
Toxic Shock Syndrome	Nafcillin 150 mg/kg/day IV div q6h x 7 days	General supportive care of prime importance
Tularemia	Gentamicin 6 mg/kg/day IM, IV div q8h OR streptomycin 30 mg/kg/day IM div q12h; x 7-10 days (Dosage of streptomycin may be reduced by 1/2 after 3 days)	Monitor serum conc of gentamicin; tetracycline less effective alternative
Typhoid fever	Chloramphenicol 50(PO)-75(IV) mg/kg/day div q6h OR amoxicillin 100 mg/kg/day PO div q8h x 14 days	TMP/SMX; ceftriaxone and cefotaxime are also effective
Varicella-Zoster, disseminated (compromised host)	Acyclovir 1500 mg/m^2/day (approx 45 mg/kg/day) IV as 1-2 hr infusion div q8h OR vidarabine 10 mg/kg/day as 6 hr IV infusion; x 5 days	Also used for severe or complicated chickenpox

2 VII. PREFERRED THERAPY FOR SPECIFIC PATHOGENS

NOTES:
1. For parasitic and fungal infections see Sections IX and VIII, respectively.
2. Resistance of nosocomial gram-negative bacilli to aminoglycosides is a common problem; therefore, the suggested aminoglycosides may not be appropriate in all situations.

Organism	Clinical Illness	Drug of Choice	Alternatives
Acinetobacter calcoaceticus	Sepsis, meningitis	Imipenem	Anti-Pseudomonas beta-lactam + amikacin; TMP/SMX
Actinobacillus actinomycetemcomitans	Abscesses, endocarditis	Ampicillin	Tetracycline (Pts >7 yrs); chloramphenicol
Actinomyces israelii	Actinomycosis	Penicillin G	Tetracycline (Pts >7 yrs); ampicillin
Aeromonas spp.	Diarrhea, sepsis, cellulitis	TMP/SMX	Aminoglycoside
Arcanobacterium haemolyticum	Pharyngitis	Erythromycin	Penicillin G; a cephalosporin
Bacillus anthracis	Anthrax	Penicillin G	Erythromycin; tetracycline (Pts >7 yrs)
Bacteroides fragilis	Peritonitis, sepsis, abscesses	Chloramphenicol; clindamycin; metronidazole for CNS infection	Cefoxitin; anti-Pseudomonas penicillins; imipenem
Bacteroides, other spp.	Pneumonia, sepsis, abscesses	Penicillin G	Ampicillin; clindamycin; chloramphenicol; erythromycin
Bordetella spp.	Pertussis	Erythromycin	Ampicillin; TMP/SMX

44

Borrelia spp.	Relapsing fever, Lyme disease	Tetracycline (Pts >7 yrs)	Penicillin G; ceftriaxone; erythromycin
Branhamella catarrhalis	See *Moraxella*		
Brucella spp.	Brucellosis	Tetracycline (Pts >7 yrs); (+ gentamicin, if severe)	Chloramphenicol; TMP/SMX; rifampin
Calymmatobacterium granulomatis	Granuloma inguinale	Tetracycline (Pts >7 yrs)	Chloramphenicol; aminoglycoside
Campylobacter spp.	Diarrhea	Erythromycin	Tetracycline (Pts >7 yrs); furazolidone
	Sepsis, meningitis	An aminoglycoside	According to *in vitro* tests
Caprocytophaga canimorsus (formerly DF-2)	Sepsis following dog bite	Penicillin G	Erythromycin; a cephalosporin
Capnocytophaga ochraceae	Sepsis, abscesses	Penicillin G	Erythromycin; cefoxitin; metronidazole
Chlamydia pneumoniae (TWAR)	Pneumonia	Tetracycline (Pts >7 yrs)	Erythromycin
Chlamydia psittaci	Psittacosis	Tetracycline (Pts >7 yrs)	Chloramphenicol
Chlamydia trachomatis	Lymphogranuloma venereum	Tetracycline (Pts >7 yrs)	A sulfonamide; erythromycin
	Urethritis, vaginitis	Tetracycline (Pts >7 yrs)	Erythromycin; sulfonamide; ampicillin

(continued on next page)

45

Organism	Clinical Illness	Drug of Choice	Alternatives
Chlamydia trachomatis (cont.)	Inclusion conjunctivitis of newborn	Erythromycin (oral)	Topical erythromycin, tetracycline or sulfonamide
	Pneumonia in infancy	Erythromycin	Ampicillin; sulfonamide
	Trachoma	Topical + oral tetracycline (Pts >7 yrs)	Topical + oral sulfonamide
Chromobacterium violaceum	Sepsis, pneumonia, abscesses	Chloramphenicol	None
Citrobacter spp.	Meningitis, sepsis	An aminoglycoside	A cephalosporin; TMP/SMX
Clostridium spp.	Tetanus, gas gangrene, sepsis	Penicillin G	Tetracycline (Pts >7 yrs); clindamycin
Clostridium difficile	Antibiotic-associated colitis	Vancomycin (oral) or metronidazole (oral)	Bacitracin (oral); Vancomycin IV
Corynebacterium diphtheriae	Diphtheria	Penicillin G (+ antitoxin)	Erythromycin
Corynebacterium haemolyticum	See *Arcanobacterium*		
Corynebacterium, JK group	Sepsis	Vancomycin	According to *in vitro* tests
Corynebacterium minutissimum	Erythrasma	Topical miconazole or clindamycin	Erythromycin
Cytomegalovirus	Pneumonia, hepatitis	Ganciclovir	Foscarnet (investigational)
Dysgonic fermenter-2	See *Capnocytophaga*		

46

Organism	Infection	Drug of Choice	Alternatives
Ehrlichia canis	Systemic illness with or without rash	Tetracycline (Pts >7 yrs)	Chloramphenicol
Eikenella corrodens	Abscesses, meningitis	Tetracycline (Pts >7 yrs)	Ampicillin; aminoglycoside
Enterobacter spp.	Sepsis, pneumonia, wound infection	Ceftriaxone; cefotaxime	An aminoglycoside; imipenem; TMP/SMX
	Urinary infection	TMP/SMX	An aminoglycoside; nitrofurantoin
Enterococcus spp.	Endocarditis, urinary infection	Ampicillin + an aminoglycoside	Vancomycin + an aminoglycoside
Erysipelothrix insidiosa	Sepsis, cellulitis, abscesses	Ampicillin (?) plus aminoglycoside	Tetracycline (Pts >7 yrs)
Escherichia coli	Urinary infection, not hospital acquired	A sulfonamide	Ampicillin; amoxicillin; a cephalosporin
	Sepsis, meningitis, pneumonia, hospital acquired urinary infection	An aminoglycoside	TMP/SMX; a cephalosporin; imipenem
Flavobacterium meningosepticum	Sepsis, meningitis	Vancomycin	An aminoglycoside; TMP/SMX
Francisella tularensis	Tularemia	Gentamicin or streptomycin	Tetracycline (Pts >7 yrs); chloramphenicol
Fusobacterium spp.	Sepsis, soft tissue infection	Penicillin G	Metronidazole; clindamycin
Gardnerella vaginalis	Genital infection	Metronidazole	Clindamycin
Haemophilus aphrophilus	Sepsis, endocarditis, abscesses	Tetracycline (Pts >7 yrs)	Ampicillin

47

Organism	Clinical Illness	Drug of Choice	Alternatives
Haemophilus ducreyi	Chancroid	Ceftriaxone (1 dose)	TMP/SMX; erythromycin
Haemophilus influenzae	Otitis media	Augmentin;erythromycin-sulfa; cefaclor;cefixime; TMP/SMX	Amoxicillin (if beta-lactamase negative)
	Meningitis, arthritis, cellulitis, epiglottitis, pneumonia	Chloramphenicol; cefuroxime; ceftriaxone; cefotaxime	Ampicillin (if beta-lactamase negative)
Herpes simplex virus	Keratoconjunctivitis	Trifluridine (topical)	Vidarabine (topical)
	Encephalitis, disseminated disease	Acyclovir	Vidarabine
Human immunodeficiency virus	AIDS, ARC	Zidovudine	Dideoxyinosine (investigational)
Influenza A virus	Influenza	Amantadine	(?) Ribavirin
Klebsiella spp.	Urinary tract infection	TMP/SMX	A cephalosporin; nitrofurantoin
	Sepsis, pneumonia, meningitis	Ceftriaxone; cefotaxime	An aminoglycoside; TMP/SMX; impenem
Legionella spp.	Legionnaire's Disease and related illnesses	Erythromycin (?) + rifampin	TMP/SMX
Leptospira spp.	Leptospirosis	Penicillin G	Tetracycline (Pts >7 yrs)
Leptotrichia buccalis	Vincent's angina	Penicillin G	Erythromycin; metronidazole; clindamycin
Listeria monocytogenes	Sepsis, meningitis	Ampicillin (?) plus aminoglycoside	TMP/SMX

Organism	Disease	Drug of choice	Alternative
Moraxella catarrhalis	Otitis, sinusitis, bronchitis	Augmentin; erythromycin + sulfa	TMP/SMX; cefixime; cefaclor
Moraxella other spp.	Bone and joint infection; abscess	Penicillin G	Ampicillin; aminoglycoside
Morganella morganii	Urinary infection, sepsis	An aminoglycoside	A cephalosporin
Mycobacterium tuberculosis	Tuberculosis	Isoniazid and rifampin (? + pyrazinamide)	Aminoglycoside; cycloserine; ethambutol; ethionamide
Mycobacteria, nontuberculous ("atypical")	Cervical adenitis	None (Surgery)	Rifampin
	Pneumonia	Rifampin and (?) amino-glycoside; rifabutin (ansamycin); clofazimine	(Variable susceptibility to antibiotics)
Mycobacterium marinum (M. balnei)	Papules, pustules, cold abscesses (Swimmer's granuloma)	(?) TMP/SMX; rifampin	None (usually self-limited)
Mycobacterium leprae	Leprosy	Dapsone + rifampin + clofazimine	
Mycoplasma hominis	Non-gonococcal urethritis	Clindamycin	Tetracycline (Pts >7 yrs)
Mycoplasma pneumoniae	Pneumonia	Erythromycin	Tetracycline (Pts >7 yrs)
Neisseria gonorrhoeae beta-lactamase negative	Gonorrhea	Amoxicillin + probenecid; ceftriaxone	Penicillin G
N. gonorrhoeae, beta-lactamase positive	Gonorrhea	Ceftriaxone; spectinomycin	TMP/SMX; other cephalosporins

49

Organism	Clinical Illness	Drug of Choice	Alternatives
Neisseria meningitidis	Sepsis, meningitis	Penicillin G	Ampicillin; chloramphenicol; A sulfonamide (if susceptible); cephalosporin
Nocardia asteroides	Nocardiosis	A sulfonamide (? amikacin initially)	Amikacin; TMP/SMX; cycloserine; erythromycin
Pasteurella multocida	Sepsis, abscesses	Penicillin G	Tetracycline; ampicillin; chloramphenicol
Peptostreptococcus	Sepsis	Penicillin G	Clindamycin; vancomycin
Plesiomonas shigelloides	Diarrhea, meningitis	TMP/SMX	Aminoglycoside
Propionibacterium acnes	Sepsis, skin lesions	Penicillin G	Tetracycline; clindamycin; erythromycin; cephalosporin
Proteus mirabilis	Urinary infection, sepsis, meningitis	Ampicillin	Aminoglycoside; TMP/SMX
Proteus, other spp.	Urinary infection, sepsis, meningitis	Cefotaxime; ceftriaxone	Imipenem; an aminoglycoside
Providencia spp.	Sepsis	Cefotaxime; ceftriaxone	TMP/SMX; imipenem; an aminoglycoside
Pseudomonas aeruginosa	Urinary infection	Anti-Pseudomonas beta-lactam	An aminoglycoside; imipenem
	Sepsis, pneumonia	Anti-Pseudomonas beta-lactam + an aminoglycoside	Imipenem

Organism	Clinical Illness	Drug of Choice	Alternatives
Pseudomonas cepacia	Pneumonia, sepsis	TMP/SMX; ceftazidime	According to in vitro tests
Pseudomonas mallei	Glanders	Tetracycline (Pts >7 yrs) + streptomycin	Chloramphenicol; gentamicin
Pseudomonas maltophilia	See *Xanthomonas maltophilia*		
Pseudomonas pseudomallei	Melioidosis	Ceftazidime OR chloramphenicol + sulfa + aminoglycoside for sepsis	TMP/SMX or tetracycline (Pts >7 yrs) for chronic disease
Respiratory syncytial virus	Bronchiolitis, pneumonia	Ribavirin	None
Rickettsia	Rocky Mountain spotted fever, Q fever, typhus, rickettsialpox, ehrlichiosis	Tetracycline (Pts >7 years)	Chloramphenicol
Salmonella spp.	Focal infections, typhoid fever, sepsis	TMP/SMX; chloramphenicol	Ampicillin; ceftriaxone
Serratia marcescens	Sepsis, pneumonia	Ceftriaxone; cefotaxime	TMP/SMX; an aminoglycoside; imipenem
Shigella spp.	Enteritis, urinary infection, vaginitis	TMP/SMX	Ampicillin; tetracycline (Pts >7 yrs); chloramphenicol
Spirillum minus	Rat bite fever (Sodoku)	Penicillin G	Tetracycline (Pts >7 yrs); aminoglycoside

51

Organism	Clinical Illness	Drug of Choice	Alternatives
Staphylococcus aureus	Skin infections	Cefadroxyl	Cloxacillin; a cephalosporin; erythromycin; Augmentin
	Pneumonia, sepsis, osteomyelitis, etc.	Nafcillin	Methicillin; oxacillin; a cephalosporin; vancomycin; clindamycin
	Infections due to penicillin-susceptible strains	Penicillin G or V	Erythromycin
Staphylococcus, coagulase negative	Sepsis, infected CNS shunts, urinary infection	Vancomycin	If susceptible: nafcillin (or related drug); (?) TMP/SMX
Staphylococcus spp., methicillin-resistant	Sepsis, focal infections	Vancomycin (?) + rifampin and/or gentamicin	TMP/SMX
Streptobacillus moniliformis	Rat bite fever (Haverhill fever)	Penicillin G	Tetracycline (Pts >7 yrs); aminoglycoside
Streptococcus, Groups A or B, anaerobic, non-enterococcal Group D	Pharyngitis, impetigo, adenitis	Penicillin V or benzathine penicillin	Erythromycin
	Pneumonia, sepsis, meningitis	Penicillin G or ampicillin	A cephalosporin; vancomycin
Streptococcus, enterococcus group	See *Enterococcus*		
Streptococcus, viridans group	Endocarditis	Penicillin G (± aminoglycoside)	Vancomycin; a cephalosporin

52

Organism	Disease	Drug of choice	Alternative
Streptococcus pneumoniae	Pneumonia, otitis	Penicillin V or G	Erythromycin; cephalosporin
	Meningitis, arthritis, sepsis	Penicillin G	Vancomycin (for penicillin-resistant strains); chloramphenicol, vancomycin, cephalosporin for relatively resistant strains
Treponema pallidum	Syphilis	Penicillin G	Tetracycline (Pts >7 yrs); erythromycin; cephalosporin
Treponema pertenue	Yaws	Penicillin G	Tetracycline (Pts >7 yrs)
Ureaplasma urealyticum	Genitourinary infections	Erythromycin	Tetracycline (Pts >7 yrs)
Varicella-Zoster virus	Disseminated disease; zoster (shingles)	Acyclovir	Vidarabine
Vibrio cholerae	Cholera	Tetracycline (Pts >7 yrs)	TMP/SMX
Vibrio vulnificus	Sepsis	Tetracycline (Pts >7 yrs)	Penicillin G
Xanthomonas maltophilia	Sepsis	Aminoglycoside (?) + rifampin	TMP/SMX; ceftazidime
Yersinia enterocolitica	Enteritis, arthritis, sepsis	? Tetracycline; TMP/SMX	? Erythromycin
Yersinia pestis	Plague	Streptomycin + chloramphenicol or tetracycline (Pts >7 yrs)	TMP/SMX; other aminoglycoside
Yersinia pseudotuberculosis	Adenitis	? Tetracycline	? TMP/SMX

VIII. ANTIFUNGAL THERAPY

Infection	Therapy	Comments
SYSTEMIC INFECTIONS		
Aspergillosis	Amphotericin B initial dose 0.25 mg/kg IV in 6 hour infusion of 0.1 mg/ml concentration in 5% dextrose sol'n (no saline). Increase daily dosage by 0.25 mg/kg increments to maximum daily (or q.o.d.) dosage of 1 mg/kg. Total dosage 30-35 mg/kg given over period of 4-6 weeks or longer. NOTE: If patients tolerate drug as 1-2 hr infusion, pain, paresthesias, etc. are of briefer duration. (For allergic bronchopulmonary aspergillosis see page 27)	Treat only for severe or disseminated forms; Monitor CBC and renal function; Interrupt therapy if abnormalities; Resume at lower dosage when values return to normal or administer less frequently. Clinical value of *in vitro* synergy bewtween amphotericin B and rifampin or flucytosine is not established.
Blastomycosis (North American)	Amphotericin B (as above) OR ketoconazole 6 mg/kg/day PO div q12-24 hr x 6 months	Treat only progressive or severe disease; Fluconazole may be effective
Candidiasis		
- Disseminated infection	Amphotericin B (as above) but daily dosage 0.5-0.75 mg/kg OR amphotericin B PLUS flucytosine 100-150 mg/kg/day PO div q6h OR fluconazole 3-6 mg/kg once daily (dosage for children not established)	Hematologic toxicity with flucytosine; Intrathecal amphotericin B for meningitis is usually not needed
- Urinary infection	Flucytosine 50-100 mg/kg/day PO div q6h x 7 days OR fluconazole (as above)	If complicates antibiotic therapy, stopping antibiotic sometimes leads to spontaneous cure.

- Esophagitis in neutropenic patients	Flucytosine 150 mg/kg/day PO div q6h OR clotrimazole 10 mg troche PO q4h x 7 days OR fluconazole (as above)	Amphotericin B if no response or for severe disease
Chromomycosis	Flucytosine OR ketoconazole (as above)	
Coccidioidomycosis	Amphotericin B (as above) OR (for non-life threatening disease) ketoconazole (as above); fluconazole may be effective	Regimen of systemic amphotericin B and ketoconazole and intrathecal miconazole for meningitis appears successful
Cryptococcosis	Flucytosine 100-150 mg/kg/day PO div q6h PLUS amphotericin B 0.3-0.5 mg/kg IV daily x 6 weeks or longer; OR fluconazole 6 mg/kg once daily (dosage for children not established)	Monitor for hematologic toxicity; Synergy permits use of lower dosage of amphotericin B
Histoplasmosis	Amphotericin B (as above) OR ketoconazole (as above); fluconazole may be effective	Ketoconazole only for chronic forms
Paracoccidioidomycosis	Ketoconazole (as above) OR amphotericin B (as above)	Sulfa drugs may be effective.
Phaeohyphomycosis	Amphotericin B (as above) x 3 wks or longer	Surgery, as necessary
Phycomycosis (Mucormycosis)	Amphotericin B (as above) x 6 wks or longer	Surgery, as necessary; Intrathecal amphotericin B may be needed for CNS infection.

55

Infection	Therapy	Comments
Pneumocystis carinii **infection**	Trimethoprim-sulfamethoxazole 20 mg TMP-100 mg SMX/kg/day IV, PO div q6h OR pentamidine isethionate 4 mg base/ kg/day IV daily x 10-14 days; trimetrexate 30 mg/m² daily + leucovorin may be effective	Prophylaxis: 5 mg TMP-25 mg SMX/kg/day once daily PO OR 300 mg aerosolized pentamidine once monthly (adult dosage; dosage for children not established)
Pseudallescheria boydii **and** *Scedosporium apiospermum* **infection**	Miconazole 20-40 mg/kg/day IV div q8h x 3 wks or longer	Fluconazole may be effective
Sporotrichosis	Sat. solution of potassium iodide 1-2 drops per year of age 3 x daily PO (maximum 30 drops t.i.d.) until lymphocutaneous lesions resolved (give with fruit juice or milk)	Amphotericin B for dissemi- nated infection

LOCALIZED MUCOCUTANEOUS INFECTIONS

Dermatophytoses

- Scalp (including kerion)	Griseofulvin microcrystalline 10-15 mg/kg once daily x 1-2 mos or longer (Taken with milk or fatty foods to augment absorption) OR ketoconazole 6 mg/kg/day div q12-24h	Topical antifungal agent does not help heal acute stage but may prevent recurrence from endothrix spores; Selsun shampoo twice weekly may be useful adjunct
- Glabrous skin, hands or feet	Topical miconazole, clotrimazole, ketoconazole or ciclopirox applied 3x daily x 7-10 days (longer for palmar/plantar infections)	
- Tinea versicolor	Selenium sulfide (Selsun) OR topical clotrimazole (or related drug) applied twice daily x 7-10 days	Recurrence common; Ketoconazole PO also provides improvement

Infection	Therapy	Comments
Candidiasis		
- Benign mucocutaneous	Topical nystatin, clotrimazole or miconazole 3-4 x daily x 7-10 days	0.5% aqueous gentian violet for refractory cases
- Oral thrush	Nystatin suspension in mouth 3-4 x daily after feedings x 7-10 days	
- Chronic mucocutaneous	Ketoconazole 6 mg/kg/day PO div q12-24h until lesions clear	Occurs in hosts with variety of immune defects
- Vulvovaginal	Miconazole (200 mg suppository) or clotrimazole (200 mg tablet) intravaginally at bedtime x 3 days	May require 7 days therapy

57

IX. ANTIPARASITIC THERAPY

Note: Familiarize yourself with the toxic potentials of these drugs and monitor the patient accordingly. For some of the parasitic diseases, drugs available only from the Centers for Disease Control are the preferred therapy. These drugs are indicated by "(CDC)". Consultation for diagnostic tests and detailed information about experimental drugs are available around the clock from the CDC and they will send drugs to you. The telephone number during the day is 404-639-3670. Nights and weekends call 404-639-2888 and ask the duty officer for the Parasitic Disease Drug Service doctor on call.

Disease/Organism	Treatment
AMEBIASIS *Entamoeba histolytica*	
- Asymptomatic carrier	Iodoquinol (formerly diiodohydroxyquin) 40 mg/kg/day (max 2g) PO div q8h x 20 days; OR diloxanide furoate (CDC) 20 mg/kg/day PO div q8h x 10 days OR paromomycin (CDC) 30 mg/kg/day PO div q8h x 7 days
- Mild to moderate colitis	Metronidazole 35-50 mg/kg/day PO div q8h x 10 days; OR paromomycin 30 mg/kg/day PO div q8h x 7 days EITHER DRUG FOLLOWED BY iodoquinol or diloxanide, as above, x 20 days
- Severe colitis	Metronidazole 35-50 mg/kg/day PO, IV div q8h x 10 days OR dehydroemetine (CDC) 1.0-1.5 mg/kg/day (max 90 mg) IM div q12h x 5 days EITHER DRUG FOLLOWED BY iodoquinol, as above, x 20 days
- Liver abscess and other extra-intestinal disease	Metronidazole, as above, x 10 days FOLLOWED BY iodoquinol, as above, x 20 days; OR dehydroemetine (CDC), as above, FOLLOWED BY chloroquine 10 mg base/kg/day PO x 14-21 days PLUS iodoquinol, as above, x 20 days
AMEBIC MENINGOENCEPHALITIS *Naegleria* spp., *Acanthamoeba* spp., *Hartmannella* spp.	Amphotericin B 1 mg/kg/day IV x uncertain duration, (?) PLUS miconazole and rifampin for *Naegleria*; Intrathecal miconazole (10 mg) daily may be helpful; Acanthamoeba susceptible *in vitro* to ketoconazole, flucytosine, pentamidine
Ancylostoma duodenale	See HOOKWORM

ANGIOSTRONGYLIASIS
Angiostrongylus spp.

Thiabendazole 50-75 mg/kg/day PO div q8h for *A. costaricensis* x 3 days OR mebendazole 100 mg PO b.i.d. x 5 days for *A. cantonensis*

ANISAKIASIS
Anasakis spp.

Removal by fibroendoscopy

ASCARIASIS
Ascaris lumbricoides

Pyrantel pamoate 11 mg/kg PO x 1 dose OR mebendazole 100 mg b.i.d. x 3

BABESIOSIS
Babesia spp.

Clindamycin (30 mg/kg/day PO div q6-8h) and quinine (25 mg/kg/day PO div q8h) x 7 days effective in limited experience; exchange blood transfusion reported helpful (Pentamidine and TMP/SMX may be effective)

BALANTIDIASIS
Balantidium coli

Metronidazole 35 mg/kg/day PO div q8h x 5-7 days OR tetracycline (Pts >7 yrs) 40 mg/kg/day PO div q6h x 10 days OR iodoquinol 40 mg/kg/day PO div q8h x 20 days

BLASTOCYSTIASIS
Blastocystis hominis

Metronidazole 35 mg/kg/day PO div q8h x 10 days OR iodoquinol 40 mg/kg/day (max 2g) PO div q8h x 20 days (Based on anecdotal reports)

CAPILLARIASIS
Capillaria philippinensis

Mebendazole 200 mg PO b.i.d. (regardless of body weight) x 20 days OR thiabendazole 25 mg/kg PO div q12h x 30 days

CHAGA'S DISEASE
Trypanosoma cruzi

See TRYPANOSOMIASIS

Clonorchis sinensis

(See FLUKES)

CRYPTOSPORIDIOSIS
Cryptosporidium parvum

No proved effective therapy; spiramycin 100 mg/kg/day PO div q12h x 10 days effective in one report

59

Disease/Organism	Treatment
CUTANEOUS LARVA MIGRANS or CREEPING ERUPTION (Cutaneous hookworm)	Thiabendazole suspension topically b.i.d. x 2-5 days; OR thiabendazole 50 mg/kg/day PO div q12h x 3 days; Note: ethylene chloride spray and carbon dioxide snow are effective but painful and sometimes damage tissue
CYSTICERCOSIS *Cysticercus cellulosae*	Surgery, when indicated; praziquantel 50 mg/kg/day div q8h x 14 days; For CNS cysticercosis give steroids starting 1 day before first dose of praziquantel; (Praziquantel therapy is controversial)
DIENTAMOEBIASIS *Dientamoeba fragilis*	Iodoquinol 40 mg/kg/day (max 2g) PO div q8h x 20 days; OR metronidazole 35 mg/kg/day PO div q8h x 7-10 days; OR tetracycline (Pts >7 yrs) 40 mg/kg/day PO div q8h x 10 days
Diphyllobothrium latum	See TAPEWORMS
DIROFILARIASIS *Dirofilaria immitis*	Surgical excision of subcutaneous or pulmonary nodules; praziquantel possibly effective
DRACUNCULOSIS *Dracunculus medinensis* (Guinea worm)	Metronidazole 25 mg/kg/day PO div q8h x 10 days; OR thiabendazole 50-75 mg/kg PO div q12h x 3 days; IN ADDITION remove worm by winding out a few cm each day
ECHINOCOCCOSIS *Echinococcus granulosus*	Surgical treatment when indicated; albendazole 10 mg/kg/day PO div q12h x 28 days
Entamoeba histolytica	See AMEBIASIS
Enterobius vermicularis	See PINWORMS
Fasciola hepatica	See FLUKES
FILARIASIS	
- River blindness *Onchocerca volvulus*	Ivermectin (CDC) 150 mcg/kg (0.15 mg/kg) PO as single dose; repeat q6mos; antihistamines or corticosteroids for allergic reactions

60

- Other forms (Loa loa, tropical eosinophilia)
Wuchereria bancrofti, Brugia malayi

Diethylcarbamazine test doses of 25 mg on Day 1, 50 mg t.i.d. on Day 2, 100 mg t.i.d. on Day 3; then 6 mg/kg/day (9 mg/kg/day for loa loa) PO div q8h x 18 days (10 days for tropical eosinophilia); antihistamines or corticosteroids for allergic reactions; surgical excision of subcutaneous nodules, preferably before drug therapy

FLUKES

- Sheep liver fluke (*Fasciola hepatica*)
- Lung fluke (*Paragonimus westermani*)
- Chinese liver fluke (*Clonorchis sinensis*) and others (*Fasciolopsis, Heterophyes, Metagonimus, Opisthorchis*)

Praziquantel 75 mg/kg PO div q8h x 1-2 days is drug of choice for all fluke infections except *F. hepatica* for which bithionol (CDC) is given (3)-50 mg/kg qod x 10-15 doses)

GIARDIASIS
Giardia lamblia

Furazolidone 8 mg/kg/day PO div q6h x 7-10 days OR quinacrine 6 mg/kg/day PO div c8h x 7 days; OR metronidazole 15 mg/kg/day div q8h x 7 days (all can have Antabuse-like effect)

GNATHOSTOMIASIS
Gnathostoma spinigerum

Surgical removal OR mebendazole 200 mg PO q3h x 6 days (regardless of body weight)

HOOKWORM
Necator americanus, Ancylostoma duodenale

Mebendazole 100 mg PO t.i.d. x 3 days (regardless of body weight); OR pyrantel pamoate 11 mg/kg PO daily x 3 days

Hymenolepis nana

See TAPEWORMS

ISOSPORIASIS
Isospora belli

Trimethoprim-sulfamethoxazole 10 mg TMP-50 mg SMX/kg/day div q6h x 10 days; then, 5 mg TMP-50mg SMX/kg/day div q12h x 3 wks

LEISHMANIASIS, including Kala Azar
Leishmania braziliensis, L. donovani, L. tropica, L. mexicana

Stibogluconate sodium (CDC) 20 mg/kg/day (max 800 mg) IM or IV, daily x 20 days (10 mg/kg/day x 10 days for *L. tropica*); ALTERNATIVES, for *L. donovani*, pentamidine isethionate 4 mg/kg/day IM daily for 14 days; OR, for *L.braziliensis* and *L. mexicana*, amphotericin B 1 mg/kg/day IV x 4-8 wks (Concomitant treatment with interferon gamma has been used for refractory cases of visceral disease)

61

Disease/Organism	Treatment
LICE *Pediculus capitis* or *humanus*, *Phthirus pubis*	Permethrim 1% (NIX Creme Rinse) OR pyrethins (RID, A-200 Pyrinate liquid or shampoo, R & C Shampoo) OR malathion 0.5% (Ovide lotion) OR lindane (Kwell) applied topically once (follow manufacturer's instructions for use); repeat in 1 wk; for eyelashes, use yellow oxide of mercury ophthalmic ointment; launder bedding and clothing
MALARIA	CDC Malaria Hotline (24 hrs a day) 404/332-4555
Prophylaxis - For areas without resistant *P. falciparum*	Chloroquine or amodiaquine 5 mg base/kg (max 300 mg) PO once weekly, beginning 1-2 weeks before arrival in malarial zone and continuing for 6 weeks after last exposure (drugs available in liquid form outside the USA); PLUS (optional) (beginning with final 2 weeks of chloroquine Rx) primaquine 0.3 mg base/kg PO daily x 14 days after departure from endemic area for individuals heavily exposed to mosquitoes
- For areas where chloroquine-resistant *P. falciparum* exists	Chloroquine (as above); Have pyrimethamine-sulfadoxine (Fansidar) available to take if febrile illness develops; OR (for adults) mefloquine 250 mg once weekly starting 1 week before travel and for 4 weeks after leaving area
Treatment of disease - *Plasmodium vivax, P. ovale*	Chloroquine 10 mg base/kg (max 600 mg) PO stat, then 5 mg base/kg at 6 hrs, 24 hrs and 48 hrs after initial dose; FOLLOWED BY primaquine 0.3 mg base/kg PO once daily x 14 days. (Note: parenteral chloroquine is available from the CDC for emergency use)
- *P. malariae*	Chloroquine (as for P. vivax)
- *P. falciparum* chloroquine-susceptible	Chloroquine (as for P. vivax)

- P. falciparum
chloroquine-resistant

Quinine 25 mg/kg/day PO div q8h x 3 days <u>AND</u> Fansidar (pyrimethamine-sulfadoxine): <1 yr, 1/4 tab; 1-3 yrs, 1/2 tab; 4-8 yrs, 1 tab; 9-14 yrs, 2 tab; >14 yrs, 3 tab as a single dose; NOTE: Several alternative regimens have been reported for Fansidar-resistant infections: quinine x 3 days + tetracycline x 7 days; quinidine 10 mg/kg q8h x 7 days; mefloquine 25 mg/kg PO as a single dose (not approved for use in children)

- P. falciparum CNS disease

Parenteral quinine (CDC) 8 mg/kg IV as 2 hr infusion; repeat doses q8h; <u>OR</u> quinidine 10 mg/kg IV loading dose, followed by 0.02 mg/kg/min (until oral quinine can be taken)

Paragonimus westermani

See FLUKES

PINWORMS
Enterobius vermicularis

Pyrantel pamoate 11 mg/kg PO x 1 dose <u>OR</u> mebendazole 100 mg PO (regardless of body weight) x 1 dose; repeat treatment in 2 weeks

PNEUMOCYSTIS PNEUMONIA
Pneumocystis carinii

See page 56

SCABIES
Sarcoptes scabei

Permethrin 5% cream applied to entire body (incl scalp in infants), left on for 8-14 hr before bathing; <u>OR</u> lindane (Kwell) lotion applied to all of body below neck, leave on overnight, bathe in AM; launder bedding and clothing; topical corticosteroid <u>after</u> treatment for persistent itching

SCHISTOSOMIASIS
Schistosoma hematobium, japonicum, mansoni, mekongi

Praziquantel 20 mg/kg PO x 2-3 doses taken in 1 day

STRONGYLOIDIASIS
Strongyloides stercoralis

Thiabendazole 50 mg/kg/day PO div q12h x 2 days (5 days or longer for disseminated disease)

TAPEWORMS

- Cysticercus cellulocae

See CYSTICERCOSIS

63

Disease/Organism	Treatment
- *Echinococcus granulosus*	See ECHINOCOCCOSIS
- *Taenia saginata, T. solium, Hymenolepis nana, Diphyllobothrium latum, Dipylidium caninum*	Niclosamide approx 40 mg/kg PO chewed thoroughly x 1 dose (for *H. nana* treat for 6 days) OR praziquantel 10-20 mg/kg x 1 dose (25 mg/kg for *H. nana*)
TOXOPLASMOSIS *Toxoplasma gondii*	Pyrimethamine 2 mg/kg/day PO div q12h x 3 days, then 1 mg/kg/day (max 25 mg every other day) PO (Supplemental folinic acid) AND trisulfapyrimidines or sulfadiazine 120 mg/kg/day PO div q6h; OR spiramycin (CDC) 50-100 mg/kg/day PO div q6h; treatment continued for 4-6 wks after resolution of illness (See page 8 for congenital toxoplasmosis)
TRICHINOSIS *Trichinella spiralis*	Anti-inflammatory drugs; steroids for CNS or severe symptoms; mebendazole 200-400 mg t.i.d. x 3 days, then 400-500 mg t.i.d. x 10 d
TRICHOMONIASIS *Trichomonas vaginalis*	Metronidazole 40 mg/kg (max 2g) PO x 1 dose; OR metronidazole 15 mg/kg/day (max 1 g/day) PO div q8h x 7 days; treat sex partners
TRICHOSTRONGYLIASIS *Trichostrongylus orientalis*	Pyrantel pamoate 11 mg/kg PO x 1 dose OR thiabendazole 50 mg/kg/day PO div q12h x 2 days
Trichuris trichiura	See WHIPWORM
TRYPANOSOMIASIS	
- **CHAGA'S DISEASE** *Trypanosoma cruzi*	Nifurtimox (CDC); obtain dosage recommendations from CDC
- **SLEEPING SICKNESS** *T. brucei gambiense; T. b. rhodesiense*	Acute stage: suramin (CDC) 20 mg/kg IV on days 1, 3, 7, 14 and 21 OR pentamidine isethionate 4 mg/kg/day IV x 10 days
	Late disease with CNS involvement: melarsoprol (CDC) initial dose 0.35 mg/kg IV, gradually increase dosage to maximum dose of 3.6 mg/kg given at 1-5 day intervals for total of 10 doses (18-25 mg/kg) over 1 month period

VISCERAL LARVA MIGRANS
Toxocara canis; T. cati

Thiabendazole 50 mg/kg/day PO div q12h x 5 days or longer; corticosteroids for severe symptoms and for eye infection; diethylcarbamazine 6 mg/kg/day div q8h x 7-10 days

WHIPWORM (TRICHURIASIS)
Trichuris trichiura

Mebendazole 100 mg PO b.i.d. (regardless of body weight) x 3 days

Wuchereria bancrofti

See FILARIASIS

X. ALPHABETICAL LISTING OF ANTIBIOTICS WITH DOSAGE FORMS AND USUAL DOSAGES

NOTES:

1. When a range of dosage is given, the higher dosages are generally indicated for serious illnesses.
2. In some cases the dosages indicated differ from the manufacturers' recommendations in the package inserts.
3. IV preparations available in ready-to-use "piggy-back" bottles are not included in the tabulated dosage forms.

Generic and Trade® Names	Dosage Form	Route	Dosage	Interval
Acyclovir Zovirax®	5% ointment	Topical	q.s. to cover lesions	q3h
	500 mg vial	IV as 1-3 hr infusion	25-50 mg/kg/day	q8h
	200 mg cap	PO	1 cap 5 times daily	q4h
Amantadine HCl Symmetrel®	100 mg cap 50 mg/5 ml syrup	PO	5-8 mg/kg/day (max. 200 mg/day)	q12h
Amikacin sulfate Amikin®	0.1, 0.5, 1 g vials	IM, IV	15-20 mg/kg/day	q8h
Aminosalicylic acid	0.5, 1 g tab; powder in 1 lb btl or 4 g pkg	PO	300 mg/kg/day	q8-12h
Amoxicillin trihydrate Amoxil®, Polymox®, Trimox®, Wymox®, generic	250, 500 mg cap 125, 250 mg/5 ml susp 50 mg/ml drops	PO	40 mg/kg/day	q8h

66

Drug	Preparation	Route	Dose	Frequency
Amoxicillin and clavulanate potassium Augmentin®	"Augmentin 125" (125 mg amox + 31.25 mg clav)/5 ml susp; also chewable tab "Augmentin 250" (250 mg amox + 62.5 mg clav)/5 ml susp; also chewable tab "Augmentin 250" (250 mg amox + 125 mg clav) tab; "Augmentin 500" (500 mg amox + 125 mg clav) tab	PO	40 mg amox component/kg/day	q8h
Amphotericin B Fungizone®	50 mg vial	IV	0.25-1 mg/kg/day	q1-2 days
Ampicillin and Ampicillin trihydrate Omnipen®, Polycillin®, Principen®, generic	250, 500 mg cap 125 mg chewable tab 125, 250, 500 mg/5 ml susp 100 mg/ml drops	PO	50 mg/kg/day	q6h
Ampicillin, sodium Omnipen®, Polycillin®, generic	0.125, 0.25, 0.5, 1, 2, 4 g vials	IM, IV	100-200 mg/kg/day (meningitis 200-400)	q6h
Ampicillin/Sulbactam Unasyn®	1 g amp/0.5 g sul, 2 g amp/1 g sul	IV	As per the ampicillin component	q6h
Azlocillin sodium Azlin®	2, 3, 4 g vials	IV	300-450 mg/kg/day (approved only for children with cystic fibrosis)	q4-6h
Aztreonam Azactam®	0.5, 1, 2 g vials	IM, IV	90-120 mg/kg/day	q6-8h
Bacampicillin HCl Spectrobid®	400 mg tab (equiv to 280 mg ampicillin) 125 mg/5 ml susp	PO	25-50 mg/kg/day	q12h

Generic and Trade® Names	Dosage Form	Route	Dosage	Interval
Bacitracin	10,000, 50,000 unit vials	IM	800-1200 u/kg/day (not recommended)	q8h
Carbenicillin, disodium Geopen®	1, 2, 5, 10 g vials	IV	400-600 mg/kg/day	q4-6h
Carbenicillin indanyl sodium Geocillin®	382 mg tab	PO	30-50 mg/kg/day	q6h
Cefaclor Ceclor®	125, 187, 250, 375 mg/5 ml susp 250, 500 mg cap	PO	40 mg/kg/day	q8-12h
Cefadroxil monohydrate Duricef®, Ultracef®, generic	500 mg cap, 1 g tab 125, 250, 500 mg/5 ml susp	PO	30 mg/kg/day	q12h
Cefamandole nafate Mandol®	0.5, 1, 2 g vials	IV, IM	100-150 mg/kg/day	q4-6h
Cefazolin sodium Ancef®, Kefzol®, Zolicef®, generic	0.25, 0.5, 1 g vials	IM, IV	50-100 mg/kg/day	q8h
Cefixime Suprax®	200, 400 mg tab 100 mg/5 ml susp	PO	8 mg/kg/day	q12-24h
Cefmetazole sodium Zefazone®	1, 2 g vials	IV	No established dosage for children	q8-12h
Cefonicid sodium Monocid®	0.5, 1 g vials	IV, IM	(?) 20-40 mg/kg/day (not approved for children)	q24h
Cefoperazone Cefobid®	1, 2 g vials	IV, IM	100-150 mg/kg/day (not approved for children)	q8-12h

68

Ceforanide lysine Precef®	0.5, 1, 2 g vials	IM, IV	20-40 mg/kg/day	q12h
Cefotaxime sodium Claforan®	0.5, 1, 2 g vials	IV, IM	100-150 mg/kg/day (meningitis 200)	q6-8h
Cefotetan Cefotan®	1, 2 g vials	IV, IM	(?) 40-80 mg/kg/day (not approved for children)	q12h
Cefoxitin sodium Mefoxin®	1, 2 g vials	IV, IM	80-160 mg/kg/day	q4-6h
Ceftazidime Fortaz®, Tazicef®, Tazidime®	0.5, 1, 2 g vials	IV, IM	100-150 mg/kg/day (meningitis 150)	q8h
Ceftizoxime sodium Cefizox®	1, 2 g vials	IV, IM	150-200 mg/kg/day	q6-8h
Ceftriaxone Rocephin®	0.25, 0.5, 1 g vials	IM, IV	50-100 mg/kg/day (meningitis 100)	q12-24h q12h
Cefuroxime Kefurox®, Zinacef®	0.75, 1.5 g vials	IV, IM	100-150 mg/kg/day (meningitis 240)	q8h q6h
Cefuroxime axetil Ceftin®	125, 250, 500 mg tab	PO	30 mg/kg/day (40 for otitis)	q12h
Cephalexin monohydrate Keflet®, Keflex®, Keftab®, generic	250, 500 mg tab 0.25, 0.5, 1 g cap 100 mg/ml drops 125, 250 mg/5 ml susp	PO	25-50 mg/kg/day	q6h
Cephalothin, sodium	1, 2, 4 g vials	IM, IV	75-125 mg/kg/day	q4-6h
Cephapirin, sodium Cefadyl®	1, 2, 4 g vials	IM, IV	40-80 mg/kg/day	q6h

69

Generic and Trade® Names	Dosage Form	Route	Dosage	Interval
Cephradine Anspor®, Velosef®, generic	250, 500 mg cap 125, 250 mg/5 ml susp	PO	25-50 mg/kg/day	q6h
	0.25, 0.5, 1 g vials	IM, IV	50-100 mg/kg/day	q6h
Chloramphenicol Chloramphenicol palmitate Chloromycetin®, generic	250 mg cap 150 mg/5 ml susp	PO	50-75 mg/kg/day (meningitis 75-100)	q6h
Chloramphenicol sodium succinate Chloromycetin®	1 g vial	IV		
Chloroquine HCl Aralen HCl®	250 mg amp (equiv to 200 mg base)	IM	5 mg base/kg	1 or 2 doses
Chloroquine PO₄ Aralen PO₄®, generic	500 mg tab (equiv to 300 mg base)	PO	10 mg base/kg/day	q24h
Chloroquine, hydroxy Plaquenil®	200 mg tab (equiv to 155 mg base)			
Cinoxacin Cinobac®	250, 500 mg cap	PO	(?) 20 mg/kg/day (not approved for children)	q6-12h
Ciprofloxacin Cipro®	250, 500, 750 mg tab	PO	20-30 mg/kg/day (not approved for children < 21 yrs)	q12h
Clindamycin HCl hydrate Clindamycin palmitate HCl	75, 150, 300 mg cap 75 mg/5 ml sol'n	PO	20-30 mg/kg/day	q6h
Clindamycin phosphate Cleocin®, generic	0.15, 0.3, 0.6 g amp	IM, IV	25-40 mg/kg/day	q6-8h

70

Drug	Form	Route	Dose	Interval
Clofazimine Lamprene®	50, 100 mg cap	PO	1 mg/kg/day	q24h
Cloxacillin, sodium Cloxapen®, Tegopen®, generic	250, 500 mg cap; 125 mg/5 ml sol'n	PO	50-100 mg/kg/day	q6h
Colistimethate, sodium Coly-Mycin M®	20, 150 mg vials	IM, IV	5-7 mg/kg/day	q8h
Colistin sulfate Coly-Mycin S®	25 mg/5 ml susp	PO	5-15 mg/kg/day	q8h
Cyclacillin generic	250, 500 mg cap	PO	50-100 mg/kg/day	q8h
Cycloserine Seromycin®	250 mg cap	PO	(?) 7-10 mg/kg/day (No recommended dosage for children)	q12h
Dapsone	25, 100 mg scored tab	PO	1 mg/kg/day	q24h
Demeclocycline HCl Declomycin®	150 mg cap; 150, 300 mg tab	PO	8-12 mg/kg/day	q6-12h
Dicloxacillin monohydrate, sodium Dycill®, Dynapen®, Pathocil®, generic	125, 250, 500 mg cap; 62.5 mg/5 ml susp	PO	12-25 mg/kg/day	q6h
Dideoxyinosine Videx®	250, 1000 g vials	IV, PO	(?) 180 mg/m²/day (Dosage for children not established)	q8h
Diiodohydroxyquin (See Iodoquinol)				
Doxycycline hyclate Doryx®, Vibramycin®, Vibra-Tabs®, generic	50, 100 mg cap	PO	2-4 mg/kg/day (Pts >7 yrs)	q12h on 1st day; then 1/2 dose q24h
Doxycycline calcium Vibramycin®	50 mg/5 ml syrup			

71

Generic and Trade® Names	Dosage Form	Route	Dosage	Interval
Doxycycline monohydrate Vibramycin®	25 mg/5 ml susp	PO	(See previous page)	
Doxycycline hyclate Vibramycin®	100, 200 mg vials	IV	2-4 mg/kg/day (Pts >7 yrs)	q24h as 2 hr infusion
Erythromycin E-mycin®, ERYC®, Ery-Tab®, Erythromycin Base Filmtab®, Ilotycin®, PCE Dispertab®, generic	125 mg pellets in cap 250 mg tab, cap 330 mg tab	PO	40 mg/kg/day	q6h
	2% topical sol'n for acne 0.5% ophthalmic ung	Topical Topical		
Erythromycin estolate Ilosone®, generic	100 mg/ml drops 500 mg tab 125, 250 mg cap 125, 250 mg chewable tab 125, 250 mg/5 ml susp	PO	30-40 mg/kg/day	q8-12h
Erythromycin ethylsuccinate E.E.S.®, EryPed®, Wyamycin E®	400 mg tab 200 mg chewable tab 200, 400 mg/5 ml susp 100 mg/2.5 ml drops	PO	40 mg/kg/day	q6h
Erythromycin ethylsuccinate and sulfisoxazole acetyl Pediazole®, Eryzole®	200 mg erythromycin and 600 mg sulfisoxazole/5 ml susp	PO	40 mg/kg/day of erythromycin component	q6-8h
Erythromycin gluceptate Ilotycin Gluceptate®	0.25, 0.5, 1 g amp	IV	20-50 mg/kg/day	contin- uous infusion; or q6h

72

Drug	Preparation	Route	Dosage	Interval
Erythromycin lactobionate Erythrocin Lactobionate®, generic	0.5, 1 g vial	IV	20-40 mg/kg/day	q6h (1-2 hr infusion)
Erythromycin stearate Erythrocin Stearate®, Wyamycin S®, generic	250, 500 mg tab	PO	20-40 mg/kg/day	q6h
Ethambutol hydrochloride Myambutol®	100, 400 mg tab	PO	15 mg/kg/day	q24h
Ethionamide Trecator-SC®	250 mg tab	PO	(?) 10-20 mg/kg/day (No established dosage for children)	q12h
Fluconazole Diflucan®	50, 100, 200 mg tab 200 mg vial	PO IV	(?) 3-6 mg/kg/day (No established dosage for children)	q24h
Flucytosine Ancobon®	250, 500 mg cap	PO	50-150 mg/kg/day	q6h
Furazolidone Furoxone®	100 mg tab 50 mg/15 ml susp (contains kaolin and pectin)	PO	5-8 mg/kg/day	q6h
Ganciclovir Cytovene®	500 mg vial	IV	Induction: 10 mg/kg/day	q12h (1-2 hr infusion)
			Maintenance: 5 mg/kg/day (No established dosage for children)	q24h
Gentamicin sulfate Garamycin®, generic	20, 80 mg vials (parenteral)	IM, IV	3-7.5 mg/kg/day (cystic fibrosis 7-10)	q8h

73

Generic and Trade® Names	Dosage Form	Route	Dosage	Interval
Gentamicin (cont.)				
Garamycin Intrathecal®	4 mg vial (intrathecal)	Intrathecal	1-2 mg/day	q24h
Griseofulvin Fulvicin P/G®, Fulvicin U/F®, Grifulvin V®, Grisactin®, Gris-PEG®	microsize: 125, 250, 500 mg tab, cap 125 mg/5 ml susp ultramicrosize: 125, 250 mg tab	PO	15 mg/kg/day	q24h
Imipenem-Cilastatin Primaxin®	250/250, 500/500 mg vials	IM, IV	60-100 mg/kg/day (not approved for children)	q6h
Iodoquinol (formerly diiodohydroxyquin) Yodoxin®	650 mg tab	PO	40 mg/kg/day	q8h
Isoniazid INH®, Laniazid®, generic	100, 300 mg scored tab 1 g vial	PO, IM	10-20 mg/kg/day (max. 300 mg)	q12-24h
Isoniazid and pyridoxine	10 mg/0.5 mg/ml syrup	PO	(See isoniazid)	
Kanamycin sulfate Kantrex®, generic	75 mg, 0.5, 1 g vials	IM, IV	15-30 mg/kg/day	q8h
	500 mg cap	PO	150-250 mg/kg/day (for suppression of bowel flora)	q1-6h
Ketoconazole Nizoral®	200 mg scored tab	PO	5-10 mg/kg/day	q12-24h
Lincomycin hydrochloride Lincocin®	250, 500 mg cap 250 mg/5 ml syrup	PO	30-60 mg/kg/day	q8h
	0.6, 3 g vials	IM, IV	10-20 mg/kg/day	q8-12h

74

Mebendazole Vermox®	100 mg chewable tab	PO	See Section IX	
Mefloquine HCl Lariam®	250 mg tab	PO	See Section IX	
Methacycline HCl Rondomycin®	150, 300 mg cap	PO	10 mg/kg/day	q6-12h
Methenamine hippurate Hiprex®, Urex®	1 g tab	PO	25-50 mg/kg/day	q12h
Methenamine mandelate Mandelamine®, Thiacide®, Uroquid®, generic	0.35, 0.5, 1 g tab 250, 500 mg/5 ml susp 0.5, 1 g granules	PO	50-75 mg/kg/day	q6h
Methicillin, sodium Staphcillin®	1, 4, 6 g vials	IM, IV	150-200 mg/kg/day	q6h
Metronidazole Flagyl®, Metric-21®, Protostat®, generic	250, 500 mg tab	PO	15-35 mg/kg/day	q8h
Mezlocillin sodium Mezlin®	500 mg vial	IV	30 mg/kg/day	q6h
	1, 2, 3, 4 g vials	IV	200-300 mg/kg/day	q4-6h
Miconazole Monistat®	200 mg amp	IV	20-40 mg/kg/day	q8h
Minocycline HCl Minocin®	50, 100 mg cap 50 mg/5 ml syrup	PO	4 mg/kg/day	q12h
	100 mg vial	IV	4 mg/kg/day	q12h (2h infusion)
Moxalactam Moxam®	1, 2 g vials	IV	150-200 mg/kg/day (meningitis 200)	q6-8h q6h

Generic and Trade® Names	Dosage Form	Route	Dosage	Interval
Mupirocin Bactroban®	15 g tube	Topical	Apply to infected skin	q8h
Nafcillin monohydrate, sodium Nafcil®, Unipen®	250 mg cap, 500 mg tab 250 mg/5 ml sol'n	PO	50-100 mg/kg/day	q6h
	0.5, 1, 2 g vials	IM, IV	150 mg/kg/day	q6h
Nalidixic acid NegGram®	0.25, 0.5, 1 g tab 250 mg/5 ml susp	PO	55 mg/kg/day	q6h
Neomycin sulfate	500 mg tab 125 mg/5 ml sol'n	PO	50-100 mg/kg/day	q6-8h
Netilmicin Netromycin®	50, 150 mg vials	IV, IM	3-7.5 mg/kg/day	q8h
Niclosamide Niclocide®	500 mg scored tab	PO	40 mg/kg/day	q24h
Nitrofurantoin Furadantin®	50, 100 mg scored tab 25 mg/5 ml susp	PO	5-7 mg/kg/day	q6h
Nitrofurantoin macrocrystals Macrodantin®, generic	25, 50, 100 mg cap	PO	5-7 mg/kg/day	q6h
Norfloxacin Noroxin®	400 mg tab	PO	400 mg (adults); (Not approved for children < 21 yrs)	q12h
Nystatin Mycostatin®, generic	100,000 u/ml susp 500,000 u tab	PO (not swallowed)	Infants 2 ml/dose; children 4-6 ml or 1 tab/dose	q6h

76

Drug	Preparation	Route	Dose	Frequency
Oxacillin, sodium Bactocill®, Prostaphlin®, generic	250, 500 mg cap 250 mg/5 ml sol'n	PO	50-100 mg/kg/day	q6h
Oxytetracycline	0.25, 0.5, 1, 2, 4 g vials	IM, IV	150-200 mg/kg/day	q6h
Oxytetracycline, calcium	125, 250 mg cap, tab 125 mg/5 ml syrup	PO	40-50 mg/kg/day	q6h
Oxytetracycline HCl	125, 250 mg cap			
Oxytetracycline HCl Terramycin®	50, 100, 250 mg vials with 2% lidocaine	IM	15-25 mg/kg/day	q8-12h
Paromomycin sulfate Humatin®	250 mg cap 125 mg/5 ml syrup	PO	30 mg/kg/day	q8h
Penicillin G, benzathine Bicillin®	3 million unit 10 ml vial; 1, 1.5 and 2 ml syringes containing 600,000 u/ml	IM	50,000 u/kg	1 dose
Penicillin G, potassium Pentids®, Pfizerpen G®, generic	125, 150, 250, 500 mg tab 125, 250, 500 mg/5 ml syrup 1, 2, 10, 20 million unit vials	PO IM, IV	25-50 mg/kg/day 100,000-250,000 u/kg/day	q6-8h q4h
Penicillin G, procaine Wycillin®	0.3, 0.6, 1.2, 2 4 million unit vial	IM	25,000-50,000 u/kg/day	q12-24h
Penicillin G, sodium	5 million unit vial	IM, IV	100,000-250,000 u/kg/day	q4h
Penicillin V Betapen-VK®, Pee Vee K®, Veetids®, generic	125, 250, 500 mg tab 125, 250 mg/5 ml sol'n 125, 250 mg/5 ml drops	PO	25-50 mg/kg/day	q6-8h

Generic and Trade® Names	Dosage Form	Route	Dosage	Interval
Pentamidine isethionate Pentam 300®, NebuPent®	300 mg vial	IV	4 mg/kg/day	q24h
Piperacillin Pipracil®	2, 3, 4 g vials	IV	200-300 mg/kg/day (Not approved for children)	q4-6h
Polymyxin B sulfate Aerosporin®	50 mg (500,000 unit) vial	IM, IV	3-4.5 mg/kg/day	q6h (IM); continous infusion (IV)
Praziquantel Biltricide®	600 mg 3-scored tab	PO	75 mg/kg	In 3 doses x 1 day
Pyrantel pamoate Antiminth®	250 mg/5 ml susp	PO	11 mg/kg	1 dose
Pyrazinamide	500 mg tab	PO	30 mg/kg/day	q12-24h
Pyrimethamine (See sulfadoxine) Daraprim®	25 mg scored tab	PO	0.5-1 mg/kg/day	q12h
Quinacrine HCl Atabrine®	100 mg tab	PO	6 mg/kg/day	q8h
Ribavirin Virazole®	6 g vial	Inhalation	1 vial by SPAG-2 aerosol generator	q24h
Rifampin Rifadin®, Rimactane®	150, 300 mg cap 600 mg vial	PO IV	10-20 mg/kg/day (max 600 mg)	q12-24h
Spectinomycin HCl Trobicin®	2, 4 g vials	IM	30-40 mg/kg	1 dose

78

Drug	Preparation	Route	Dosage	Interval
Streptomycin sulfate	1, 5 g vials	IM	20-30 mg/kg/day	q12h
Sulfadiazine	0.3, 0.5 g tab	PO	120-150 mg/kg/day	q4-6h
Sulfadiazine, sodium	2.5 g amp	SC, IV	100 mg/kg/day	q6-8h
Sulfadoxine and pyrimethamine Fansidar®	500 mg SDX + 25 mg PMA scored tab	PO	(See Section IX)	
Sulfamethizole Thiosulfil®	0.25, 0.5 g tab 0.25 g/5 ml susp	PO	30-45 mg/kg/day	q6h
Sulfamethoxazole Gantanol®, generic	0.5, 1 g tab 0.5 g/5 ml susp	PO	50-60 mg/kg/day	q12h
Sulfasalazine Azulfidine®, generic	500 mg tab	PO	30-60 mg/kg/day	q4-8h
Sulfisoxazole Gantrisin®, generic	0.5 g tab 0.5 g/5 ml susp or syrup	PO	120-150 mg/kg/day	q4-6h
Tetracycline Achromycin®, Sumycin®, generic	250, 500 mg cap, tab 125 mg/5 ml syrup 125, 250 mg/5 ml susp	PO	25-50 mg/kg/day	q6h
	250, 500 mg vials 250, 500 mg vials	IM IV	15-25 mg/kg/day 20-30 mg/kg/day	q8-12h q8-12h (2h infusion)
Thiabendazole Mintezol®	500 mg chewable, scored tab 500 mg/5 ml susp	PO	50 mg/kg/day	q12h
Ticarcillin disodium Ticar®	1, 3, 6 g vials	IV	200-300 mg/kg/day	q4-6h

79

Generic and Trade® Names	Dosage Form	Route	Dosage	Interval
Ticarcillin and clavulanate potassium Timentin®	3/0.1, 3/0.2 g vials	IV	200-300 mg/kg/day (not approved for children)	q4-6h
Tobramycin sulfate Nebcin®, generic	20, 80, 1.2 g vials	IV, IM	3-6 mg/kg/day (cystic fibrosis 7-10)	q8h
Trifluridine Viroptic®	1% ophthal. sol'n	Topical	1 drop	q2h
Trimethoprim Proloprim®, Trimpex®, generic	100 mg scored tab	PO	4 mg/kg/day (not approved for children <12 yrs)	q12h
Trimethoprim-Sulfamethoxazole Bactrim®, Septra®, generic	80 mg TMP/400 mg SMX tab 160 mg TMP/800 mg SMX tab 40 mg TMP/200 mg SMX/5 ml susp	PO	6-12 mg TMP/ 30-60 mg SMX/kg/day; (20 mg TMP/100 mg SMX/kg/day for *Pneumocystis*)	q12h
	400 mg TMP/2000 mg SMX amp	IV		q6h
Troleandomycin Tao®	250 mg cap 125 mg/5 ml susp	PO	25-40 mg/kg/day	q6h
Vancomycin HCl Vancocin®, Vancoled®	1 g bottle 125, 250 mg cap	PO	10-50 mg/kg/day	q6h
Vancor®, generic	500 mg vial	IV	40 mg/kg/day (meningitis 60)	q6h
Vidarabine Vira-A®	3% ophthalmic ointment	Topical	Approx 1 cm of ointment	q3h
	1 g vial	IV	10-30 mg/kg/day	q24h
Zidovudine Retrovir®®	100 mg cap 50 mg/5 ml syrup	PO	See page 39	q6h

XI. ALPHABETICAL LISTING OF TRADE NAMES

[**Trade Name** (Drug Company)--Generic Name]

- A -

Achromycin (Lederle)
--Tetracycline

Aerosporin (Burroughs Wellcome)
--Polymyxin B

Amikin (Bristol Myers Squibb)
--Amikacin

Amoxil (SmithKline Beecham)
--Amoxicillin

Ancef (SmithKline Beecham)
--Cefazolin

Ancobon (Roche)
--Flucytosine

Anspor (SmithKline Beecham)
--Cephradine

Antiminth (Pfizer)
--Pyrantel pamoate

Aralen (Winthrop)
--Cloroquine

Aralen with Primaquine (Winthrop)
--Cloroquine/primaquine

Atabrine (Winthrop)
--Quinacrine

A/T/S (Hoechst-Roussel)
--2% erythromycin sol'n (Topical)

Augmentin (SmithKline Beecham)
--Amoxicillin/clavulanate potassium

Aureomycin (Lederle)
--Chlortetracycline (Topical)

Azactam (Bristol Myers Squibb)
--Aztreonam

Azlin (Miles)
--Azlocillin

Azo Gantanol (Roche)
--Sulfamethoxazole/phenazopyridine

Azo Gantrisin (Roche)
--Sulfisoxazole/phenazopyridine

Azulfidine (Pharmacia)
--Sulfasalazine

- B -

Bacitracin (Quad)
--Bacitracin

Bactrim (Roche)
--Trimethoprim/sulfamethoxazole

Bactroban (SmithKline Beecham)
--Mupirocin (Topical)

Bactocill (SmithKline Beecham)
--Oxacillin

Benemid (Merck Sharp & Dohme)
--Probenecid

Betapen VK (Bristol Myers Squibb)
--Penicillin V

Bicillin (Wyeth Ayerst)
--Benzathine penicillin G

Biltricide (Miles)
--Praziquantel

- C -

Ceclor (Lilly)
--Cefaclor

Cefadyl (Bristol Myers Squibb)
--Cephapirin

Cefizox (LyphoMed)
--Ceftizoxime

Cefobid (Roerig)
--Cefoperazone

Cefotan (Stuart)
--Cefotetan

Ceftin (Allen & Hanburys)
--Cefuroxime axetil

Chloromycetin (Parke-Davis)
--Chloramphenicol

Cinobac (Dista)
--Cinoxacin

Cipro (Miles)
--Ciprofloxacin

Claforan (Hoechst-Roussel)
--Cefotaxime

Cleocin (Upjohn)
--Clindamycin
Cloxapen (SmithKline Beecham)
--Cloxacillin
Coly-Mycin (Parke-Davis)
--Colistin
Cytovene (Syntex)
--Ganciclovir

- D -

Dapsone USP (Jacobus)
--Dapsone
Daraprim (Burroughs Wellcome)
--Pyrimethamine
Declomycin (Lederle)
--Demeclocycline
Diflucan (Roerig)
--Fluconazole
Doryx (Parke-Davis)
--Doxycycline
Duricef (Mead Johnson)
--Cefadroxil
Dycill (SmithKline Beecham)
--Dicloxacillin
Dynapen (Bristol Myers Squibb)
--Dicloxacillin

- E -

E. E. S. (Abbott)
--Erythromycin ethylsuccinate
Elimite cream (Herbert)
--Permethin 5% (Topical)
E-Mycin (Upjohn)
--Erythromycin
ERYC (Parke-Davis)
--Erythromycin
EryDerm (Abbott)
--2% erythromycin sol'n (Topical)
EryPed (Abbott)
--Erythromycin ethylsuccinate
EryTab (Abbott)
--Erythromycin
Erythrocin Lactobionate (Abbott)
--Erythromycin lactobionate
Erythrocin Stearate (Abbott)
--Erythromycin stearate

Erythromycin Base Filmtab (Abbott)
--Erythromycin
Erythromycin Stearate (P-D/Lederle)
--Erythromycin stearate
Eryzole (Alra)
--Erythromycin ethylsuccinate/
sulfisoxazole acetyl

- F -

Fansidar (Roche)
--Sulfadoxine/pyrimethamine
Flagyl (Searle)
--Metronidazole
Fortaz (Glaxo)
--Ceftazidime
Fulvicin (Schering)
--Griseofulvin
Fungizone (Bristol Myers Squibb)
--Amphotericin B
Furacin (Norwich Eaton)
--Nitrofurazone (Topical)
Furadantin (Norwich Eaton)
--Nitrofurantoin
Furoxone (Norwich Eaton)
--Furazolidone

- G -

Gantanol (Roche)
--Sulfamethoxazole
Gantrisin (Roche)
--Sulfisoxazole
Garamycin (Schering)
--Gentamicin
Geocillin (Roerig)
--Carbenicillin indanyl
Geopen (Roerig)
--Carbenicillin disodium
Grifulvin V (Ortho)
--Griseofulvin
Grisactin (Wyeth Ayerst)
--Griseofulvin
Gris-PEG (Herbert)
--Griseofulvin

- H -

Hiprex (Merrell Dow)
--Methanamine hippurate
Humatin (Parke-Davis)
--Paromomycin

- I -

Ilosone (Dista) .
--Erythromycin estolate
Ilotycin (Dista)
--Erythromycin
Ilotycin Gluceptate (Dista)
--Erythromycin gluceptate
INH (Ciba)
--Isoniazid
Isoniazid (Lilly; Danbury)
--Isoniazid

- K -

Kantrex (Bristol Myers Squibb)
--Kanamycin
Keflet (Dista)
--Cephalexin
Keflex (Dista)
--Cephalexin
Keflin (Lilly)
--Cephalothin
Keftab (Dista)
--Cephalexin
Kefurox (Lilly)
--Cefuroxime
Kefzol (Lilly)
--Cefazolin

- L -

Lamprene (Geigy)
--Clofazimine
Laniazid (Lannett)
--Isoniazid
Lariam (Roche)
--Mefloquine
Lincocin (Upjohn)
--Lincomycin
Lotrimin (Schering)
--Clotrimazole (Topical)

- M -

Macrodantin (Norwich Eaton)
--Nitrofurantoin
Mandelamine (Parke-Davis)
--Methenamine mandelate
Mandol (Lilly)
--Cefamandole
Mefoxin (Merck Sharp & Dohme)
--Cefoxitin
Metric-21 (Fielding)
--Metronidazole
Mezlin (Miles)
--Mezlocillin
Minocin (Lederle)
--Minocycline
Mintezol (Merck Sharp & Dohme)
--Thiabendazole
Monistat (Ortho; Janssen)
--Miconazole
Monocid (SmithKline Beecham)
--Cefonicid
Moxam (Lilly)
--Moxalactam
Myambutol (Lederle)
--Ethambutol
Mycelex (Miles)
--Clotrimazole
Mycitracin (Upjohn)
--Neomycin/bacitracin (Topical)
Mycostatin (Bristol Myers Squibb)
--Nystatin
Mysteclin-F (Bristol Myers Squibb)
--Tetracycline/amphotericin B

- N -

Nafcil (Bristol Myers Squibb)
--Nafcillin
Nebcin (Dista)
--Tobramycin
NebuPent (LyphoMed)
--Pentamidine aerosol
NegGram (Winthrop)
--Nalidixic acid
Neosporin (Burroughs Wellcome)
--Neomycin, polymyxin B (Topical)

Netromycin (Schering)
--Netilmicin
Niclocide (Miles)
--Niclosamide
Nix Creme Rinse (Burroughs Wellcome)
--Permethrim 1% (Topical)
Nizoral (Janssen)
--Ketoconazole
Noroxin (Merck Sharp & Dohme)
--Norfloxacin

- O -
Omnipen (Wyeth Ayerst)
--Ampicillin
Ovide Lotion (GenDerm)
--Malathion 0.5% (Topical)

- P -
Pathocil (Wyeth Ayerst)
--Dicloxacillin
PCE Dispertab (Abbott)
--Erythromycin particles in tablets
Pediazole (Ross)
--Erythromycin ethylsuccinate/
sulfisoxazole acetyl
Pentam 300 (LyphoMed)
--Pentamidine isethionate
Pentids (Bristol Myers Squibb)
--Penicillin G
PenVee K (Wyeth Ayerst)
--Penicillin V
Pfizerpen (Roerig)
--Penicillin G
Pipracil (Lederle)
--Piperacillin
Plaquenil (Winthrop)
--Hydroxychloroquine
Polycillin (Bristol Myers Squibb)
--Ampicillin
Polymox (Bristol Myers Squibb)
--Amoxicillin
Polysporin (Burroughs Wellcome)
--Polymyxin B/bacitracin (Topical)
Polytrim Ophthalmic Solution (Allergan)
--Trimethoprim and polymyxin B
(Topical)

Precef (Bristol Myers Squibb)
--Ceforanide
Primaxin (Merck Sharp & Dohme)
--Imipenem-cilastatin
Principen (Bristol Myers Squibb)
--Ampicillin
Proloprim (Burroughs Wellcome)
--Trimethoprim
Prostaphlin (Bristol Myers Squibb)
--Oxacillin
Protostat (Ortho)
--Metronidazole
Pyrazinamide (Lederle)
--Pyrazinamide

- R -
Retrovir (Burroughs Wellcome)
--Zidovudine
Rifadin (Merrell Dow)
--Rifampin
Rifamate (Merrell Dow)
--Rifampin/isoniazid
Rimactane (Ciba)
--Rifampin
Rimactane/INH Dual Pack (Ciba)
--Rifampin/isoniazid
Rocephin (Roche)
--Ceftriaxone
Rondomycin (Wallace)
--Methacycline

- S -
Septra (Burroughs Wellcome)
--Trimethoprim/sulfamethoxazole
Seromycin (Lilly)
--Cycloserine
Sodium Sulamyd (Schering)
--Sodium sulfacetamide (Topical)
Spectrobid (Roerig)
--Bacampicillin
Staphcillin (Bristol Myers Squibb)
--Methicillin
Streptomycin (Roerig)
--Streptomycin
Sumycin (Bristol Myers Squibb)
--Tetracycline

Suprax (Lederle)
--Cefixime
Symmetrel (DuPont)
--Amantadine

- T -

Tao (Roerig)
--Troleandomycin
Tazicef (SmithKline Beecham)
--Ceftazidime
Tazidime (Lilly)
--Ceftazidime
Tegopen (Bristol Myers Squibb)
--Cloxacillin
Terramycin (Roerig)
--Oxytetracycline
Thiacide (Beach)
--Methenamine mandelate
Thiosulfil (Ayerst)
--Sulfamethizole
Ticar (SmithKline Beecham)
--Ticarcillin
Timentin (SmithKline Beecham)
--Ticarcillin/clavulanate
Tinactin (Schering)
--Tolnaftate (Topical)
Topicycline (Norwich Easton)
--Tetracycline (Topical)
Trecator-SC (Wyeth Ayerst)
--Ethionamide
Trimox (Bristol Myers Squibb)
--Amoxicillin
Trimpex (Roche)
--Trimethoprim
Trobicin (Upjohn)
--Spectinomycin

- U -

Ultracef (Bristol Myers Squibb)
--Cefadroxil
Unasyn (Roerig)
--Ampicillin/sulbactam
Unipen (Wyeth Ayerst)
--Nafcillin
Urex (Riker)
--Methenamine hipprate

Urobiotic (Roerig)
--Oxytetracycline, sulfamethizole/
phenazopyridine
Uroquid-Acid (Beach)
--Methenamine/sodium acid phosphate

- V -

Vancocin (Lilly)
--Vancomycin
Vancoled (Lederle)
--Vancomycin
Vancor (Adria)
--Vancomycin
Veetids (Bristol Myers Squibb)
--Penicillin V
Velosef (Bristol Myers Squibb)
--Cephradine
Vermox (Janssen)
--Mebendazole
Vibramycin (Roerig, Pfizer)
--Doxycycline
Vibra-Tabs (Pfizer)
--Doxycycline
Videx (Bristol Myers Squibb)
--Dideoxyinosine
Vioform (Ciba)
--Iodochlorhydroxyquin (Topical)
Vira-A (Parke-Davis)
--Vidarabine
Virazole (ICN)
--Ribavirin
Viroptic (Burroughs Wellcome)
--Trifluridine (Ophthalmic)

- W -

Wyamycin E (Wyeth Ayerst)
--Erythromycin ethylsuccinate
Wyamycin S (Wyeth Ayerst)
--Erythromycin stearate
Wycillin (Wyeth Ayerst)
--Penicillin G procaine
Wymox (Wyeth Ayerst)
--Amoxicillin

- Y -

Yodoxin (Glenwood)
--Iodoquinol (formerly
diiodohydroxyquin)

- Z -

Zefazone (Upjohn)
--Cefmetazole
Zinacef (Glaxo)
--Cefuroxime
Zolicef (Bristol Myers Squibb)
--Cefazolin
Zovirax (Burroughs Wellcome)
--Acyclovir

XII. ANTIBIOTIC THERAPY IN PATIENTS WITH RENAL FAILURE

Most antimicrobials are excreted primarily by the kidneys; therefore, when significant renal functional impairment is present, either downward adjustments in dosages must be made or the intervals between doses must be lengthened. Exceptions are drugs such as chloramphenicol that are metabolized to antibiotically-inactive conjugates and those excreted primarily by the liver, such as nafcillin.

Degrees of dosage adjustment necessary for treating patients with renal failure are as follows: Major adjustments in dosage and dosing intervals are necessary for treating renal failure patients with aminoglycosides, flucytosine and vancomycin. No adjustments in dosage are necessary in the use of amphotericin B, cefoperazone, chloramphenicol, cloxacillin, dicloxacillin, doxycyline, erythromycin, isoniazid, metronidazole, menocycline, nafcillin and rifampin. For other antibiotics minor to moderate adjustments are necessary. For details, see **Pocket Manual of Drug Use in Clinical Medicine**, 4th ed, by D. Craig Brater, 1989. Publisher: B.C. Decker, Inc.

The most satisfactory way to use drugs in children with decreased renal function, is by monitoring the antibiotic concentrations in serum. The customary initial loading dose is given. Initially, until antibiotic assay results are available, one makes estimates of appropriate dosage based on past experience of rates of excretion related to the degree of renal failure. Three or four serum specimens are collected at intervals over a 12-48 hour period (depending on the drug and the degree of renal failure). The serum half-life is estimated. The interval of dosing is every three half-lives for patients with moderate renal dysfunction and every two half-lives for those with severe renal failure; subsequent dosages are two-thirds or one-half, respectively, of the initial loading dose.

Patients undergoing dialysis need additional doses after the procedure if a substantial amount of drug is removed by dialysis. With peritoneal dialysis < 10% of drug is removed in the case of most antibiotics. The exceptions are aminoglycosides (20-25%), cefazolin and cefuroxime (20%), moxalactam and vancomycin (15-20%).

Removed by Hemodialysis	Beta-lactams	Other drugs
> 50%	Many cephalosporins (see exceptions below), imipenem	Acyclovir, aminoglycosides, flucytosine, isoniazid, spectinomycin, sulfonamides, trimethoprim
20 - 50%	Most penicillins (see exceptions below), aztreonam cefaclor, ceforanide, cefapirin, moxalactam	Ethambutol, metronidazole, vancomycin
< 10%	Cefixime, cefonicid, cefoperazone, cefotetan, cloxacillin, dicloxacillin, methicillin, nafcillin, oxacillin	Amphotericin B, fluoroquinolones, macrolides, miconazole, polymyxins, tetracyclines

Notes: 1. Manufacturers' recommendations for dilution of antibiotics for
intravenous use sometimes are not appropriate for pediatric patients
because of volumes of fluid that are unsuitably large for the desired time
of infusion. The dilutions given below should result in convenient
volumes, and they are well-tolerated in terms of not causing irritation of
veins.

2. The volumes of fluid in the tubing between the "piggy-back" and
the patient is approximately 15 ml. Therefore, in small babies who have
slow rates of infusion, there may be a considerable delay before the
antibiotic solution reaches the patients. It is recommended that either
(a) the antibiotic solution be injected retrograde into the tubing via a
three-way stopcock, or (b) that 10-15 ml of fluid be withdrawn from the
tubing to allow antibiotic in the "piggy-back" to enter the tubing.

3. Check the manufacturer's instructions for compatible I.V.
solutions.

Antibiotics	Recommended Final Concentration for Administration	Usual Duration of Infusion
Penicillin G	Infants: 50,000 u/ml Large Child: 100,000 u/ml	10-20 min
Aztreonam	20 mg/ml	10-20 min
Other beta-lactam antibiotics	50 mg/ml	10-20 min
Chloramphenicol	50-100 mg/ml	10-20 min
Amikacin, clindamycin, kanamycin, lincomycin	6 mg/ml	15-30 min
Gentamicin, netilmicin, tobramycin	2 mg/ml	15-30 min
Vancomycin, imipenem	5 mg/ml	60 min
Metronidazole	5-8 mg/ml	60 min
Trimethoprim-sulfamethoxazole	0.64 TMP-3.2 SMX/ml (5 ml amp in 125 ml D5W)	60 min
Vidarabine	0.45 mg/ml	12-24 hr
Acyclovir, ganciclovir	7 mg/ml	1-3 hr
Amphotericin B	0.1 mg/ml	2-6 hr

XIV. MAXIMUM DOSAGES FOR LARGE CHILDREN

Infants and young children have a large volume of distribution of many antibiotics in the body. This means that, in order to achieve good serum concentrations, we give larger doses based on body weight or surface area than are given to adults. The following dosages of commonly used drugs should not be exceeded except in unusual circumstances. (See p. 7 for oral therapy of serious infections.)

Maximum Daily Dosage	Antimicrobials
ORAL FORMULATIONS	
4-8 g	Sulfisoxazole, trisulfapyrimidines
2-3 g	Amoxicillin, ampicillin, carbenicillin, cephalexin, cephradine, chloramphenicol, cloxacillin, cyclacillin, lincomycin, nafcillin, oxacillin, penicillin G or V, tetracycline
1-2 g	Cefaclor, cefuroxime axetil, ciprofloxacin, clindamycin dicloxacillin, erythromycin, metronidazole
0.5-1.2 g	Trimethoprim
400 mg	Cefixime
PARENTERAL FORMULATIONS	
30-40 g	Carbenicillin
18-24 g	Azlocillin, mezlocillin, piperacillin, ticarcillin
10-12 g	Ampicillin, cefotaxime, ceftizoxime, cephalothin, methicillin, moxalactam, nafcillin, oxacillin
6-8 g	Aztreonam, ceftazidime
4-6 g	Cefamandole, cefoperazone, cefazolin, cefuroxime,
2-4 g	Chloramphenicol, clindamycin, erythromycin, metronidazole, spectinomycin, vancomycin
1-2 g	Amikacin, cefonicid, ceforanide, ceftriaxone, streptomycin, tetracycline
0.75-1 g	Kanamycin, lincomycin
300 mg	Gentamicin, netilmicin, tobramycin
20 million units	Penicillin G
4.8 million units	Penicillin G, procaine
2.4 million units	Penicillin G, benzathine

XV. DOSAGES BASED ON BODY SURFACE AREA

Antibiotic dosages calculated on the basis of body weight are not always appropriate for obese and malnourished patients. (Obese patients would have excessively high serum concentrations, and malnourished patients would have lower than desired serum concentrations.) For such patients dosages calculated from body surface area are preferred.

Calculation of body surface area (**J Pediatr** 93:62, 1978)

B.S.A. (m^2) = wt $(kg)^{0.5378}$ x ht $(cm)^{0.3964}$ x 0.024265, which can be solved using logarithms on a pocket calculator as:

log B.S.A. = log wt x 0.5378 + log ht x 0.3964 + log 0.024265

Antibiotics (IM or IV)	Each Dose/m^2	Interval	Amt/m^2/24 hrs
Aminoglycoside			
Amikacin, Kanamycin	200 mg	q8h	600 mg
Gentamicin, Netilmicin,			
Tobramycin	60 mg	q8h	180 mg
Beta-Lactams			
Penicillin G (meningitis)	1,750,000 u	q4h	10,500,000 u
Penicillin G (others)	450,000 u	q4h	2,700,000 u
Ampicillin, Methicillin,			
Oxacillin, Cephalothin	1.4 g	q6h	5.6 g
Ceftriaxone	1.4 g	q12h	2.8 g
Ceftazidime, Moxalactam	1.4 g	q8h	4.2 g
Nafcillin, Cefamandole,			
Cefotaxime, Ceftizoxime	1.05 g	q6h	4.2 g
Cefazolin, Cefuroxime	0.8 g	q8h	2.4 g
Cefonicid, Ceforanide	0.55 g	q12h	1.1 g
Carbenicillin	4 g	q6h	16 g
Ticarcillin, Azlocillin,			
Mezlocillin, Piperacillin	2.5 g	q6h	10 g
Aztreonam	0.8 g	q6h	3.2 g
Imipenem	0.55 g	q6h	2.2 g
Miscellaneous			
Chloramphenicol (meningitis)	0.7 g	q6h	2.8 g
Chloramphenicol (others)	0.45 g	q6h	1.8 g
Metronidazole	280 mg	q8h	840 mg
(Sulfamethoxazole	0.5 g	q8h	1.5 g)
(Trimethoprim	100 mg	q8h	300 mg)
Vancomycin (CNS infection)	0.425 g	q6h	1.7 g
Vancomycin (others)	0.275 g	q6h	1.1 g
Zidovudine	160 mg	q6h	640 mg

XVI. ADVERSE REACTIONS TO ANTIMICROBIAL AGENTS

It is a good rule of clinical practice to be suspicious of a drug reaction when a patient's clinical course deviates from the expected. This section focuses on reactions that require close observation or laboratory monitoring either because of their frequency or because of their severity. For detailed listings of reactions, consult the package inserts.

Beta-Lactam Antibiotics. The most feared reaction to penicillins, anaphylactic shock, is extremely rare and there is no absolutely reliable means of predicting its occurrence. The commercially available skin testing material, benzylpenicilloylpolylysine (Pre Pen®), should be used in conjunction with the Minor Determinant Mixture (MDM) and penicilloic acid skin testing, but the latter two are not yet commercially available. A dilute solution of penicillin G (10,000 u/ml) can be used as a skin test material in place of MDM. If the scratch test and intradermal test with 0.01 ml are negative, penicillin of the same lot number should be used for administration to the patient. (Be prepared to treat anaphylaxis.) If there is question about the allergic status one can use a desensitization schedule. (See Section III.) The monobactam, aztreonam, does not exhibit cross-sensitization with penicillins and cephalosporins.

Ampicillin and other aminopenicillins cause minor adverse effects frequently. Oral or diaper area candidiasis, diarrhea and morbilliform, blotchy "ampicillin rashes" are common. The latter is not allergic in origin and is not a contraindication to subsequent use of ampicillin or of any other penicillin. Diarrhea is somewhat less common with amoxicillin, bacampicillin and cyclacillin and slightly more common with Augmentin®. Rarely beta-lactams cause serious, life-threatening pseudomembranous enterocolitis due to suppression of normal bowel flora and overgrowth with *Clostridium difficile*. Drug fever is probably more common with ampicillin than with other penicillins. Serum sickness is uncommon. Pancytopenia is rare and reversible neutropenia and thrombocytopenia occasionally occur with any of the beta-lactams.

Nephrotoxicity is probably most common with methicillin (approximately 5%) but has been reported with all the penicillins (rarest with nafcillin). Laboratory monitoring should be performed. Hemorrhagic cystitis occurs mainly in poorly hydrated patients receiving large dosages and is probably a direct irritant effect of the large concentrations of drug in urine. It disappears even with continued use of the antibiotic when the patient's urine output increases. Carbenicillin and ticarcillin interfere with platelet function but generally do not cause clinical bleeding problems. Hypokalemia is more common with these drugs than with other beta-lactams. The ureidopenicillins (azlocillin and mezlocillin) and piperacillin appear to have similar adverse effects to carbenicillin and ticarcillin with the exception that mezlocillin has the least effect on platelet function.

Imipenem-cilastatin has similar adverse effects to other beta-lactams. In addition, patients occasionally have CNS reactions (convulsions, hallucinations, altered affect).

The cephalosporins for oral use are generally better tolerated than the penicillins. Cephaloridine has the greatest potential for nephrotoxicity. (It has been removed from the U.S. market.) The cephalosporins can cause a direct Coombs' reaction in the blood but this is of no known clinical significance. Most cephalosporins are painful on IM injection and can cause phlebothrombosis with IV administration. Cefazolin and cefuroxime are better tolerated IM and cefamandole and cephradine appear to cause fewer problems on IV use than the others. Cefaclor has been associated with a transient serum sickness-like reaction (rash, arthralgia); the cause is unknown. Similarly, a serum sickness-like reaction has been reported with IV use of cephapirin. Moxalactam, cefoperazone and cefamandole can cause a disulfiram (Antabuse)-like effect; patients should avoid alcohol, including elixirs. Prolonged prothrombin time and bleeding episodes have been attributed to the same three drugs. It is treatable (and probably preventable) with vitamin K. The third generation cephalosporins cause profound alteration of normal flora on mucosal surfaces and all have caused pseudomembranous colitis on rare occasions. Ceftriaxone commonly causes loose stools but it is rarely severe enough to require stopping therapy. Ceftriaxone can cause sludging in the gallbladder which on occasion causes symptoms and jaundice; this is reversible after stopping the drug. Ceftriaxone is also reported to displace bilirubin from albumin-binding sites.

Aminoglycosides. Any of the aminoglycosidic aminocyclitol antibiotics can cause serious nephrotoxicity and ototoxicity. (The closely related aminocyclitol, spectinomycin, is safer in this respect.) The newer aminoglycosides (amikacin, tobramycin, gentamicin and netilmicin) are generally safer than kanamycin, streptomycin or neomycin. In animal studies, netilmicin is the least ototoxic. Monitor all patients receiving aminoglycoside therapy for renal toxicity with periodic urinalyses and determinations of the BUN and creatinine and be alert to ototoxicity. It is common practice to measure the serum concentration one-half to one hour after a dose to make sure one is in a safe and therapeutic range and a trough serum concentration immediately preceding a dose. Monitoring is especially important in patients with any degree of renal insufficiency. Elevated trough concentrations (>2 μg/ml for gentamicin, netilmicin and tobramycin and >10 μg/ml for amikacin and kanamycin) should be avoided. Aminoglycosides potentiate botulinum toxin.

The "loop" diuretics (ethacrynic acid, furosemide, piretanide and bumetanide) potentiate the ototoxicity of the aminoglycosides. The "non-loop" diuretics (hydrodiuril, mercuhydrin and mannitol) do not interact with aminoglycosides to produce ototoxicity.

The aminoglycosides are well tolerated via intramuscular and intravenous routes of administration. Minor side effects such as rashes, drug fever, etc. are rare.

Chloramphenicol. The most feared toxicity of chloramphenicol, irreversible aplastic anemia, is very rare. It has been said that aplastic anemia is more likely with oral than with parenteral chloramphenicol, but it is hard to document that claim and it is probably incorrect. Regardless of the route of administration, laboratory monitoring for hematologic toxicity should be carried out in all patients treated with chloramphenicol. Transient pharmacologic bone marrow depression occurs in almost all patients receiving large dosages (> 75 mg/kg/day) of chloramphenicol. As long as the absolute neutrophil count remains more than 1,500 per μl and the platelet count above 100,000 per μl one can continue to administer chloramphenicol if it is necessary. These hematologic changes reverse rapidly when the drug is stopped.

The "gray syndrome" with fatal circulatory collapse is due to excessive accumulation of chloramphenicol in neonates secondary to delayed conjugation (because of inadequate glucuronyl transferase activity) and poor renal excretion of unconjugated chloramphenicol. Chloramphenicol should not be used in neonates unless there are no suitable alternative drugs; dosage must be restricted and, ideally, one would monitor serum concentrations (therapeutic range 10-25 μg/ml). Phenobarbitol induces glucuronidative enzymes so that patients receiving phenobarbitol may require larger than normal doses of chloramphenicol. Rifampin has a similar effect. Concomitant phenytoin administration often causes accumulation of chloramphenicol in serum which may reach toxic concentrations; conversely, accumulation of phenytoin to toxic concentrations has also been reported. Other drugs metabolized by the liver, such as theophylline, acetaminophen and isoniazid could have similar effects.

Minor side effects such as nausea and diarrhea are rare. With prolonged use (principally in children with cystic fibrosis), optic neuritis and peripheral neuritis have occurred. Alteration of normal respiratory and gastrointestinal flora may lead to infection with opportunistic bacteria or fungi. Drug fever is rare.

Tetracyclines. Tetracyclines should be used infrequently in pediatric patients because the legitimate applications are uncommon diseases (rickettsial infections, brucellosis), with the exception of acne and chlamydial infections in teenagers. Side effects include minor gastrointestinal disturbances, photosensitization, angioedema, browning of the tongue, glossitis, pruritis ani, and exfoliative dermatitis. The diarrhea associated with tetracycline administration may be a direct irritant effect or due to alteration of normal GI flora with overgrowth of opportunistic bacteria or fungi. Alterations in normal respiratory tract flora produced by tetracycline increase the risk of superinfections by staphylococci and other opportunistic organisms.

Toxic effects from tetracyclines involve virtually every organ system. Hepatic and pancreatic injury have occurred with accidental overdosage and in patients with renal failure. (Pregnant women are particularly at risk for hepatic injury.) Tetracyclines are deposited in growing bones and teeth with depression of linear bone growth and dental staining and defects in enamelization in deciduous and permanent teeth. This effect is dose-related and the risk extends up to 8 years of age. Patients taking outdated, degraded tetracycline can develop a Fanconi renal syndrome. Pseudotumor cerebri of unknown cause has rarely been seen in young infants who receive normal therapeutic doses. Minocycline causes dose-related vestibular toxicity in adults. Tetracycline is painful and irritative when injected into muscle and thrombophlebitis occurs if the drug is given IV too rapidly.

Erythromycin, Clindamycin and Lincomycin. Erythromycin is one of the safest antimicrobial agents. It commonly produces nausea and epigastric distress at dosages greater than 40 mg/kg/day. Decreased hearing which returns to normal after discontinuation of the drug has been reported several times. Alteration of normal flora is generally not a problem but oral or perianal candidiasis occasionally develops. Transient cholestatic hepatitis is a rare complication that occurs with approximately equal frequency among the various formulations of erythromycin, but the estolate poses a particular risk to pregnant women. Intramuscular administration of erythromycin is painful and irritative. IV doses should be administered slowly (1-2 hr).

Clindamycin and lincomycin can cause nausea, vomiting and diarrhea. Pseudomembranous colitis due to suppression of normal flora and overgrowth of *Clostridium difficile* is uncommon, especially in children, but potentially serious. It can be successfully treated with oral vancomycin. Urticaria, glossitis, pruritis and skin rashes occur occasionally. Serum sickness, anaphylaxis and photosensitivity are rare as are hematologic and hepatic abnormalities.

Polymyxins. Polymyxin B and polymyxin E (colistin sulfate and colistimethate) are mainly of historical interest and are rarely used now except in topical preparations. With parenteral administration the major toxicity is to the kidneys. They also cause various neurological reactions such as flushing, dizziness, ataxia, diplopia, dysphagia, and paresthesias. Neuromuscular blockade with respiratory arrest has occurred. Hematologic or hepatic toxicity has rarely been attributed to the polymyxins. Oral colistin sulfate is well tolerated with few side effects.

Antituberculous Drugs. Of the many antituberculous drugs only isoniazid, rifampin, aminosalicylic acid and the aminoglycosides are approved for use in children. Gastrointestinal irritation is very common with aminosalicylic acid. Hypersensitivity reactions such as drug fever, skin rashes and arthralgias are relatively common. Hepatic and renal toxicity is rare as are various hematologic abnormalities. Prolonged treatment with aminosalicylic acid can produce goiter. Isoniazid is generally well tolerated and hypersensitivity reactions are rare. Peripheral neuritis (preventable or reversed by pyridoxine administration) and mental aberrations from euphoria to psychosis occur more often in adults than in children. Mild elevations of ALT in the first weeks of therapy which disappear with continued administration are common. Rarely, frank hepatitis develops. Rifampin also can cause hepatitis; it is more common in patients with pre-existing liver disease or in those taking large dosages. Risk of hepatic damage increases when rifampin and isoniazid are taken together in dosages more than 15 mg/kg of each daily. Gastrointestinal, hematologic and neurologic side effects of various types have been observed on occasion. Hypersensitivity reactions are rare. Pyrazinamide can cause hepatic damage which appears to be dose-related.

Antifungal Drugs. Amphotericin B, flucytosine, miconazole and ketoconazole can produce serious adverse reactions. Amphotericin B is probably the most toxic antimicrobial drug in clinical use. Chills, fever, flushing and headaches are the commonest of the many adverse reactions. Some degree of decreased renal function occurs in up to 80% of patients given amphotericin B. Anemia is common and, rarely, hepatic toxicity and neutropenia occur.

Flucytosine is available only as an oral preparation. The major toxicity is bone marrow depression and this seems to occur mainly in patients with a pre-existing hematologic disorder and in those treated with irradiation or cancer chemotherapeutic drugs. Mild gastrointestinal upset, mental confusion and vertigo sometimes occur. Renal function should be monitored.

There is little experience with the parenteral preparation of miconazole in children but it appears to be only slightly less toxic than amphotericin B. Patients receiving miconazole should be monitored for hematologic, hepatic and renal toxicity.

Ketoconazole has produced hepatic damage on rare occasions. The most common side effect is gastric distress; this can often be alleviated by dividing the daily dose. Gynecomastia is not rare in adult males.

Fluconazole is generally well tolerated. Gastrointestinal symptoms, rash and headache occur occasionally. Transient, asymptomatic elevations of hepatic enzymes have been reported.

Vancomycin. Vancomycin can cause phlebitis if the drug is injected rapidly or in concentrated form. Vancomycin is said to have the potential for ototoxicity and nephrotoxicity, but it is difficult to document these effects in children. It was reported that vancomycin potentiated the nephrotoxicity of aminoglycosides but further study showed that this was incorrect. Hepatic toxicity is rare. Neutropenia has been reported. If the drug is infused too rapidly (fewer than 30 minutes) a transient rash of the upper body with itching may occur ("redman syndrome"). It is not a contraindication to continued use and is less likely if the infusion rate is at least 60 minutes.

Sulfonamides and Trimethoprim. The commonest adverse reaction to sulfonamides is a hypersensitivity rash. Rarely, Stevens-Johnson syndrome occurs; it was most common with very long-acting sulfas that are no longer marketed. The frequency and types of reactions to the trimethoprim-sulfamethoxazole combination are said to be the same as with sulfamethoxazole alone, but it is not clear whether Stevens-Johnson syndrome is caused more often by the combination than by sulfamethoxazole alone. Neutropenia and anemia occur rarely. The rash caused by TMP/SMX appears to be more common in patients taking large dosages. Rash is common in adults with AIDS. Mild depression of platelet counts occurs in approximately one-half the patients treated with sulfas or trimethoprim-sulfamethoxazole but this rarely produces clinical bleeding problems. Sulfa drugs can precipitate hemolysis in patients with glucose-6-phosphate dehydrogenase deficiency. Crystalline aggregates of sulfa drugs may be deposited in the kidneys or ureters and cause acute nephropathy (most likely with sulfadiazine and least likely with trisulfapyrimidines). Adequate urine output and alkalinization of the urine minimize the risk. Drug fever and serum sickness are infrequent hypersensitivity reactions. Hepatitis with focal or diffuse necrosis is rare.

Fluoroquinolones. All quinolone and fluoroquinolone drugs cause cartilage damage in toxicity studies in various immature animals, although there are no conclusive data indicating similar toxicity in young children. Studies are underway to evaluate this, but until those results are available there has been reluctance to use the fluoroquinolones in pediatric patients. Reported side effects include gastrointestinal symptoms, dizziness, headaches, tremors, confusion, seizures and rash.

XVII. ADVERSE INTERACTIONS OF DRUGS

Antibiotic	Interacting Drug	Adverse Effect
Acyclovir	Probenecid	Poss incr acyclovir toxicity
Amantadine	Anticholinergics	Hallucinations, nightmares, confusion
Amikacin (See Aminoglycosides)		
Aminoglycosides	Amphotericin B	Incr nephrotoxicity
	Anti-Pseudomonas penicillins (if renal failure)	Decr aminoglycoside effect
	Cephalosporins	Poss incr nephrotoxicity
	Digoxin	Poss decr digoxin effect
	Ethacrynic acid, furosemide, bumetanide	Incr ototoxicity
	Methotrexate	Poss incr methotrexate toxicity
	Neuromuscular blocking agents; magnesium sulfate	Incr neuromuscular blockage
Amphotericin B	Aminoglycosides	Incr nephrotoxicity
	Curariform drugs	Incr curariform effect
	Digitalis drugs	Incr digitalis toxicity
	Miconazole	Decr anti-Candida effect
	Neuromuscular blocking agents	Hypokalemia
Ampicillin	Oral contraceptives	Decr contraceptive effect
	Allopurinol	Incr incidence of rash
Cephalosporins	Alcohol (cefamandole, cefoperazone, moxalactam)	Antabuse-like effect
	Aminoglycosides	Poss incr nephrotoxicity
	Ethacrynic acid, furosemide	Incr nephrotoxicity
	Aspirin, heparin (moxalactam)	Poss incr bleeding risk

Antibiotic	Interacting Drug	Adverse Effect
	Anticoagulants (moxalactam)	Incr anticoagulant effect
Chloramphenicol	Acetaminophen	Incr chloramphenicol toxicity
	Barbiturates	Incr barbiturate effect; Decr chloramphenicol effect
	Dicumarol	Incr anticoagulant effect
	Phenytoin	Altered pharmacology of both drugs
	Rifampin	Decr chloramphenicol effect
Clindamycin, Lincomycin	Neuromuscular blocking agents	Incr neuromuscular blockade
	Diphenoxylate-atropine	Incr diarrhea, colitis
Cycloserine (See Isoniazid)		
Erythromycin	Anticoagulants	Incr anticoagulant effect
	Digoxin	Incr digoxin effect
	Theophylline	Incr theophylline effect
Furazolidone	Alcohol	Antabuse-like effect
	Alpha-adrenergic amines	Incr hypertensive effect
Gentamicin (See Aminoglycosides)		
Griseofulvin	Oral anticoagulants	Decr anticoagulant effect
	Phenobarbitol	Decr griseofulvin effect

Antibiotic	Interacting Drug	Adverse Effect
Isoniazid	Aluminum antacids	Decr isoniazid effect
	Anticoagulants	Poss incr anticoagulant effect
	Carbamazepine	Incr toxicity of both drugs
	Cycloserine	Dizziness, drowsiness
	Phenytoin	Incr phenytoin toxicity
	Rifampin	Incr hepatotoxicity
Kanamycin (See Aminoglycosides)		
Ketoconazole	Antacids	Decr ketoconazole effect
	Cimetidine	Decr ketoconazole effect
Lincomycin (See Clindamycin)		
Metronidazole	Alcohol	Antabuse-like reaction
	Anticoagulants	Incr anticoagulant effect
	Phenobarbital	Decr metronidazole effect
Miconazole (See Amphotericin B)		
Nalidixic acid	Oral anticoagulants	Incr anticoagulant effect
Netilmicin (See Aminoglycosides)		
Quinacrine	Alcohol	Antabuse-like effect

Antibiotic	Interacting Drug	Adverse Effect
Rifampin	Anticoagulants, barbiturates, beta-adrenergic blockers, contraceptives, corticosteroids, diazepam, digitoxin, hypoglycemics, quinidine	Decreased effect of interacting drug
	Chloramphenicol	Decr chloramphenicol effect
	Isoniazid	Incr hepatotoxicity
	Methadone	Methadone withdrawal symptoms
Spectinomycin	Lithium	Incr lithium toxicity
Streptomycin (See Aminoglycosides)		
Sulfonamides	Oral anticoagulants	Incr anticoagulant effect
	Hypoglycemics	Incr hypoglycemia
	Methotrexate	Poss incr methotrexate toxicity
	Phenytoin	Incr phenytoin effect
	Thiopental	Incr thiopental effect
Tetracyclines	Antacids, bismuth subsalicylate, Iron, zinc sulfate	Decr tetracycline effect
	Phenytoin, barbiturates and carbamazepine	Decr doxcyline effect
	Oral contraceptives	Decr contraceptive effect
	Lithium	Incr lithium toxicity
Thiabendazole	Theophylline	Incr theophylline effect
Tobramycin (See Aminoglycosides)		
Trimethoprim-sulfamethoxazole	Anticoagulants	Incr anticoagulant effect
	Cyclosporine	Incr nephrotoxicity
Troleandomycin	Carbamazepine	Incr carbamazepine effect
	Oral contraceptives	Jaundice
	Theophylline	Incr theophylline effect
Vidarabine	Allopurinol	Incr vidarabine toxicity

XVIII. INDEX OF DISEASES

Note: Only diseases are indexed. For alphabetical listings of microorganisms, antibiotics and trade names see Sections VII, X and XI, respectively.

NOTES

NOTES